Overcoming Common Problems

Reducing Your Risk of Cancer
What you need to know

DR TERRY PRIESTMAN

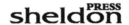

First published in Great Britain in 2008

Sheldon Press
36 Causton Street
London SW1P 4ST

Copyright © Dr Terry Priestman 2008

British Library Cataloguing-in-Publication Data
A catalogue record for this book is available from the British Library

ISBN 978-1-84709-021-8

1 3 5 7 9 10 8 6 4 2

Typeset by Fakenham Photosetting Ltd, Fakenham, Norfolk
Printed in Great Britain by Ashford Colour Press

Produced on paper from sustainable forests

Contents

Note: This is not a medical book and is not intended to replace advice from your doctor. Do consult your doctor if you are experiencing symptoms with which you feel you need help.

Introduction

Current figures predict that one in three of us will get cancer at some time during our lives. This gloomy statistic is offset by the fact that the cure rate for cancer is improving all the time, and most people who get the disease will make a full recovery. Even so, the best thing would be never to have cancer in the first place. So, how can we reduce our risk?

The single biggest risk factor for cancer is age. The older we get, the more likely we are to get it. More than three out of four cancers occur in people over the age of 65. As more of us are living longer, cancer is becoming commoner: it is one of the prices we pay for our increasing longevity. So, dying young is probably the most effective way of reducing our chances of getting the disease, but this is a rather drastic solution. In this book we'll explore some more practical, and positive, options.

The first two chapters cover some of the background, looking at what we mean by risk and how it's measured, followed by a description of some key facts about cancer. We then go on to look at different causes of cancer, and what we can do to reduce our chance of getting it, how we can move the odds in our favour. After touching on some of the many myths and falsehoods about what might cause cancer, we go on to talk about the possibility of using vaccines or drugs to prevent cancer, and the importance of screening, to look for the disease when it is at an early stage or before it even develops. Finally, there is a chapter summarizing what each of us can do to help reduce our own risk.

My aim in writing this book has been to present the evidence and offer advice. Whether or not you choose to take some, or any, of that advice is obviously entirely your choice – but my hope is that having read this book you will at least be able to make an informed decision.

Terry Priestman

To Pat Gavin
With thanks for her invaluable contribution to the care of
people in the Black Country with cancer, over the last 30 years

1

What are the risks? What is the evidence?

Introduction

Over the last 50 years medical scientists have learnt a great deal about the causes of cancer. But there are very few things, if any, that can be guaranteed to make a cancer develop. In almost every situation where something has been linked to a particular cancer, it makes it more likely that the cancer will occur but does not make it a certainty: people who smoke 50 cigarettes a day are much more likely to get lung cancer than non-smokers, but even though they have a 40 times greater chance of getting the disease, there will still be some heavy smokers who will live to a great age without ever developing it. There is no way of saying for certain which of us will, or will not, get cancer. But what we can say is that these days we know a lot of things that make it more likely that someone might get cancer, things that increase the risk. And risk is something that we will talk about a lot in this book. So before looking at cancer itself, and its causes and the things we can do to try and reduce our chances of getting it, we'll start by looking at what we mean by 'risk', and how this has been measured in scientific studies investigating the causes of different cancers.

Risk

Risk is the possible harm that could come from something we do: that harm may never happen, but there is a chance that it could. If I go on a train journey there is a risk I could be killed in a train crash; if I go out in a storm there is a risk I could be killed by lightning. In many situations the degree of risk can be worked out; the chances of something bad happening can be predicted in advance. (The risk of being killed in a railway accident is about one in 500,000; the risk of being struck by lightning is about one in 10 million.) But even when there is good scientific evidence for the risks of doing something, we often have difficulty in understanding what the numbers mean. This is partly because of a problem in clearly communicating the basic information about risk, and partly because of our inbuilt reaction to that information, our individual interpretation of what the risk means to us.

We can use words to describe the risk of something happening. But words mean different things to different people. If I tell you that I am recommending a treatment that has a high risk of you losing your hair, you may think a high risk means a 50 per cent chance (where 50 out of every 100 people would lose their hair), whereas I may think a high risk means a 90 per cent chance. We could try a different approach and use numbers: I could tell you that with the treatment 90 people out of every 100 are likely to lose their hair, but sometimes – especially in a stressful situation, which many medical consultations can be – it is easy to get confused by figures, and you still might not understand what I mean.

One possible solution is to combine words and numbers, and the European Commission Pharmaceutical Committee attempted to do this in its guidelines in 1998. These were intended to describe the risk of getting side effects from a particular treatment. The words used, along with the actual likelihood of something happening, were:

Very common	(more than 10%)	more than 1 in 10
Common	(1–10%)	1 in 100 to 1 in 10
Uncommon	(0.1–1%)	1 in 1,000 to 1 in 100
Rare	(0.01–0.1%)	1 in 10,000 to 1 in 1,000
Very rare	(less than 0.01%)	less than 1 in 10,000

But research suggested that even when given this information, people tended to overestimate their likelihood of getting side effects and were more worried than they needed to be.

Another way of getting the message across is visually, with graphs or diagrams, and one of the best methods for this is a pie chart, which many people find gives them a clear and simple view of the possible hazard in question (see Figure 1).

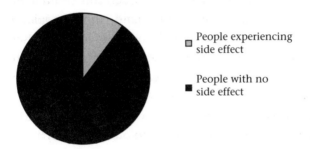

People experiencing side effect

People with no side effect

Figure 1   Pie chart showing 10 per cent risk of experiencing a side effect

Alternatively, we could use comparisons. For example, if I tell you that the chances of getting unpleasant sickness and vomiting with a particular drug are very small you may not be that reassured, but if I say that the likelihood of getting sickness with the treatment is the same as the likelihood that you will be struck by lightning on your way home, you may feel happier about taking the drug.

It is important to remember that there are two sides to risk. When we say there is a 1 per cent risk of something happening, a one in 100 chance, it also means that there is a 99 per cent chance that it won't happen. The bad news is that there is a risk, although it is only small; the good news is that 99 times out of 100, everything will be all right.

When we have got all the information – the facts, the figures, the charts and graphs, the comparisons – we then make our own decisions on what they all mean to us. We form our own judgements, and those judgements are coloured by our personal experience and things like our cultural background, religious beliefs, the opinions of family and friends, and countless other influences. If we go back to the example of hair loss: for some people this is a devastating prospect, and I have certainly looked after patients who have refused the recommended treatment for their cancer because of the risk of losing their hair, opting for a second-best approach even though this could reduce their chance of a cure. On the other hand, some people are completely unworried at the thought of being bald, and happily go ahead with treatment. In both situations the risk of hair loss is the same, but what that risk means to the individual is totally different.

Hair loss and its importance is a very personal emotion, but there can be more general aspects to our perceptions. One of my medical students recently did a survey which included quite a number of health professionals as well as members of the public, asking various questions about their views on cancer. One of the results that surprised me was that more than half the people questioned thought that regular use of mobile phones increased the risk of getting cancer. This has been the subject of a lot of research and, so far at least, there is no good evidence that this is the case. But there is a strong public perception that there is a link.

And again, even when the risks are well known, the facts are well established and the general public clearly does understand the hazards, patterns of behaviour don't always change. The most obvious example is cigarette smoking, where despite all the evidence of the harm it does and the knowledge that more than nine out of ten lung cancers are directly smoking-related, about three out of ten people still smoke, and, even more worrying, the number of young women who are smoking is on the increase.

In forming our personal ideas about risks, the experiences of people we know can be very powerful influences. If you have a close friend who has had radiotherapy for his or her cancer, and you then find out that one of your relatives is going to have radiotherapy, you will almost certainly think about what happened to your friend and use that information to understand what will happen to your relative, even though their actual treatments may be very different. This personalized, anecdotal view is almost inevitable, but it can be very misleading. To get a true picture of the risks and benefits of anything in life, we have to step back and look at large numbers of people, not just our immediate experience. For example, if 100 people were blindfolded and told to walk across a busy motorway the sad truth is that most would be run over, but just once in a while there would be a lull in the traffic and perhaps just one out of those 100 people might cross safely. Now if you happened to know that one person and he told you how he had survived the motorway crossing without injury, it wouldn't mean that walking blindfold across the M1 is perfectly safe – it would simply mean that you had met one very lucky individual. In just the same way we can't rely on what just one, or even a few, people tell us about their experience of something as being a true reflection of the overall risks and benefits involved.

Coming back to the issue of how risk is communicated, there is an important technical point to be aware of, and that is the difference between absolute risk and relative risk. Absolute risk is the chance of a particular unpleasant event occurring; relative risk is the change in that chance due to other factors. For instance, suppose for every million people, each year one person will develop a cancer of the little finger, then the risk of getting cancer of your little finger is one in a million. Clever researchers then show that among people who eat a tin of pears every day, the number of cancers of the little finger rises to two in a million. Therefore, the chances of getting cancer of your little finger are still incredibly remote, but the relative risk has actually doubled, from one in a million to two in a million. Another way of putting it is that your risk has gone up by 100 per cent. This sounds terrible and easily gives the impression that everyone will get cancer of the little finger, but in reality the risk remains almost non-existent. This means that when figures are given as relative risks they can often sound much more alarming than they really are. But giving results in this way is much more likely to grab the attention of journalists and the media, and to make a good story. As a result, the newspapers and magazines will often carry headlines about things that could double or treble your risk of a particular cancer, when in fact the real risk, the absolute risk, remains unbelievably small.

What is the evidence?

Every day the charity Cancerbackup copy me in on their press cuttings service, sending me details of all the stories relating to cancer which have appeared in the national press. At least once a week there will be a report of new research showing that something can either increase or reduce our risk of getting cancer. And this is just in the newspapers. If you add in magazines, TV, radio and, of course, the internet, the mass of information out there on what might give you cancer, or prevent it happening, is phenomenal – and often highly unreliable and misleading.

When I was a young boy my parents took the *Daily Express*. Reading the paper was an essential part of the day's routine for both of them, and they trusted it absolutely. I was brought up to believe that if it was in the *Express*, then it was the gospel truth. When I was about 12 or 13 an enlightened English master asked each of us in my class to bring a copy of yesterday's newspaper to our next lesson. We then compared and contrasted their coverage of a few of the major stories. I was amazed at the differences of opinion, emphasis and even factual content. To take just one example: whether or not the UK should join the European Union was a big issue in those days. The *Daily Express* was passionately opposed, predicting doom and disaster if we threw our lot in with foreigners, but there were other papers saying it was the only way forward and would ensure a prosperous future for us all. In an instant I developed a healthy scepticism for what the papers said: they could be informative, they could be interesting, they could be amusing, but they weren't necessarily to be believed in every detail.

The point of this story is that in order to make decisions in our lives we rely on information and experience from different sources. It may be what we read in the papers or see on the TV, what friends or relatives tell us, what we find on the internet, or what our religious beliefs dictate – the list of influences is endless. But at the end of the day we do make decisions, which may be as trivial as what to eat for breakfast or as important as whether to change job or move house. Those decisions don't just happen: they are influenced, consciously or unconsciously, by all sorts of things from different parts of our life and experience. When it comes to deciding what to believe about what might increase our chances of getting cancer or help us avoid the disease, the same applies. The information out there is infinite; choosing what is true, and what to do about it, is a process unique to each of us as individuals. The randomness, the uncertainty and the variability of this sort of decision-making is a very human thing; it happens because we are people, not machines. At first sight it may also seem to conflict with the hard facts of scientific research. If the evidence is there in learned journals from major universities or research institutes, why do we ignore it or deny it?

But how good is that evidence? The answer is that the quality of scientific research is very variable: some is excellent, but much is near to useless. Medical research is an industry: countless investigators need to make a living, literally thousands of medical and scientific journals need articles from those investigators in order to survive, universities need grants to support their investigative work – the pressure to produce and publish is immense. But when it comes to the studies on what might cause or prevent cancer, the range of the work that can be done is huge and varies enormously in quality and reliability.

The most reliable information comes from really large epidemiological surveys where carefully selected groups of (usually) thousands of people are followed up for ten or 20 years. These are extremely complex and costly pieces of work and, by definition, take decades to produce results. At the other end of the scale is an experiment, where someone takes a chemical – say, for example, a protein found in cashew nuts – and feeds it in massive doses to laboratory mice for a month, finding that they develop cancers of their left forefoot. They rush into print with a paper showing that cashew nuts cause cancer. The work is essentially meaningless as far as human cancer is concerned, and of no scientific worth, but it gets the investigator a publication, it gets the journal an article and, given the media's obsession with cancer, the likelihood is that it will get column inches around the world as a new scare story of yet another thing we should avoid if we don't want to die of cancer.

In the 1970s I was working on the development of a drug called interferon. At the time this was very newsworthy and I was interviewed for the ITV programme *World in Action*. Just before we began recording, the reporter said, 'Look, Doc, what we want is the story, not the science, OK?' I obviously didn't get it right because they never broadcast my rather downbeat assessment of the drug's prospects, in favour of other researchers who were happy to hail it as a probable cure for cancer.

By and large, unlike the media, doctors will look for the science and not the story. In recent years this approach has been more clearly set out by establishing a hierarchy and order of reliability for medical evidence. Top of the tree comes the meta-analysis – a survey which looks at the results of all available clinical trials and critically reviews their results. Then come the results of trials where patients have been randomly allocated to different treatments or procedures and the results compared (randomized controlled clinical trials). The level of importance, and worth, cascades downwards until, near the bottom of the pile, come the views of individual experts based on their personal experience – opinion-based, rather than evidence-based, medicine.

When scientific or medical studies are reported by the media they will very seldom actually mention how reliable the study is – whether the 'evidence' that some particular foodstuff might cause cancer comes from a sophisticated meta-analysis of several large, well-conducted epidemiological surveys, or is the result of a one-off experiment on ten mice in an obscure university laboratory. It is quite common not to even mention the source of the information, and certainly very rare to get an actual reference so that you could, if you wanted to, go and check on the information for yourself. What you get is the story, not the science.

Before rounding off this chapter there is one other thing I want to come back to: the difference between individuals and populations, and the power – and danger – of the anecdote. Let me explain.

A recent paper in the journal *Cancer* surveyed a group of men who had been offered the choice between surgery and radiotherapy as treatment for their early prostate cancer. They were given detailed information by their specialists, and this was backed up by booklets and leaflets giving further explanations of the pros and cons of treatment. In due course they made their decisions. The researchers then interviewed the men to see what had influenced their choice of treatment. In general the choices were based not on the scientific medical facts but on pre-existing beliefs, the views of friends or relatives, or past experience that was often inappropriate, with comments like 'I must have surgery because you can only cure cancer by cutting it out', or 'I'll have radiation because I'm terrified of the knife', or 'My mother's breast cancer was cured by surgery, so I must have an operation', and so on. A key feature of this study was the very high importance that the men interviewed gave to the individual experiences of people they knew – if a friend or family member had had radiotherapy or surgery, then what had happened to him or her played strongly in the man's own choice of treatment, even though it probably bore no relationship to his particular situation.

Looking at individuals can be very misleading. I know a man of 82 who has smoked 20 cigarettes a day since he was a teenager, and never developed lung cancer. But I don't believe that he is living proof that smoking doesn't cause cancer – he's just unbelievably lucky. The evidence from numerous studies, involving hundreds of thousands of people, is overwhelming: more than 95 per cent of lung cancers are due to smoking. There are exceptions to every rule, and once in a while you will come across a lifelong smoker who appears quite healthy. But that person's survival does not mean that smoking is good for you.

When making decisions about our health, we often look to our immediate experience, people we know, to help form our opinions, like the men in the prostate cancer study. But drawing on this very tiny evidence base can be misleading. What happens to a single individual doesn't necessarily reflect the likely outcome for a large number of people. In other words, there is no reason to believe that what happened to that person will happen to you.

Where does all this leave us?

The point of this chapter has been to try and show how difficult it is to get reliable evidence about what does, or does not, cause or prevent cancer. Most sources of information are at best unreliable. You might be lucky and get a newspaper article or internet posting that gets it just right, but often the story will distort the science, or the author's prejudices will influence the presentation. Even when you go to original published scientific literature, the quality of the work is very variable and you have to be something of an expert to know how reliable the data are. Generally speaking, a single study, a single experiment, is going to be fairly doubtful in its value: it may be right but it may be wrong, and it should always be backed up by further studies to reinforce the initial findings.

It is perfectly possible to pick up a learned medical–scientific journal and read a paper by respected investigators from a leading university or medical school, clearly showing that eating more vegetables reduces our risk of bowel cancer, and then, a month later, to see another equally learned journal, with equally respected investigators from another major institution, reporting that a vegetable-rich diet has no effect on our chances of getting bowel cancer. Neither research team is lying or falsifying their findings: it is just that this sort of epidemiological research has many pitfalls. There are a number of ways of doing these studies but none of them is perfect, and the methodology to produce a foolproof trial in this area of medicine has yet to be invented. The current solution to this dilemma is to put our faith in numbers: studies based on populations of hundreds of thousands of people are likely to give more reliable results than those involving just a few hundred subjects. In the same way, the more studies that come out with similar conclusions, the more likely it is that they are right. This is why doctors these days put such faith in meta-analyses – detailed surveys which pool the results of all the studies done on a particular subject – and use their combined findings to reach a balanced view of what may, or may not, be the truth.

Which takes me back to the real message of this section: it is unwise to put faith in any single medical or scientific report. It could be giving the definitive answer, but it is only when it has been backed up by other work reaching similar conclusions that you can really begin to believe the results. And if such carefully planned and meticulously carried out peer-reviewed research, vetted by independent experts, still needs corroboration from other similar studies in order to become accepted fact, then countless internet articles and individual anecdotes claiming to know the real truth have to be taken with a generous pinch of salt, however well-meaning or passionately convinced their authors may be. We certainly shouldn't look to anecdotes to colour our thinking. 'My story', however persuasively and emotively told, is only that, the experience of an individual, and does not reliably reflect the general picture – Mrs Jones may be absolutely certain that having eaten 20 prunes a day for the last 30 years has stopped her getting a brain tumour, but that doesn't mean she's right.

2

What is cancer?

Knowing the enemy

Up until about 20 years ago cancer was a taboo subject. People tried to avoid speaking about it, and doctors often hid the real truth from their patients, using words like 'polyps' or 'warts' to describe their malignant tumours. Telling someone what was really wrong with them was the exception rather than the rule. As a young doctor in the late 1960s I remember the panic that followed in one of our oncology outpatient clinics when an elderly lady, with a very loud voice, looked around at her fellow patients and boomed out to the receptionist, 'You wouldn't think all these people had cancer, they look quite well.'

All this secrecy and censorship left most people with little or no knowledge about cancer, and as a result fear and ignorance bred countless myths and misunderstandings. Here are three stories from my own medical days, to illustrate my point.

A few years ago I was visiting the Christie Hospital in Manchester. Running late, I took a taxi from the station. On the way the driver said, 'You'll not believe this, but at Christie's there's doctors who say they can cure cancer. Did you ever hear the like? Everyone knows you can never cure a cancer.' On another occasion I was talking to a young woman whose mother had just died and had to broach the sensitive question of whether she would want a cremation or a burial. She looked at me with some surprise. 'Why, Doctor, it'll have to be a cremation. How else can you stop the cancer growing?' And as little as ten years ago one of my patients had been admitted to a side room on a general medical ward before he could be transferred to the oncology unit. I learnt that when the patient was moved the ward sister had the side room thoroughly disinfected 'so that no one can catch the cancer'.

Cancer can be cured, cancers don't continue to grow after someone dies, and you can't 'catch' a cancer ... but given that for most of the twentieth century people tried not to speak about the condition and were given virtually no reliable information about it, it is hardly surprising that superstitions and misconceptions coloured everyone's beliefs. Despite the change in the culture and the availability of so much more information over the last couple of decades, the long shadows of the age of ignorance still linger. So this chapter is an attempt to give a scientific, unemotional account of just what cancer is, so that we can then go on to talk about how to reduce your chances of getting it.

Cancer is all about cells and genes

Each of us began our lives as a single cell – a fertilized egg in our mother's womb. That cell then divided into two new cells, those two divided to make four, the four became eight ... we had started to grow. Some nine months later we were a newborn baby, made up of more cells than there are people in the world.

From birth to adulthood we carry on growing, getting taller, broader and heavier, with the number of cells in our bodies increasing all the time. Bigger people will have more cells than smaller people, and the final number will be somewhere between 10 trillion and 100 trillion (a trillion is a million million). Numbers this huge are hard to grasp, but a trillion seconds is more than 3,000 years, and a trillion inches is almost 16 million miles.

Even when we seem to stop growing, in our late teens, cell growth keeps on going. This is because cells are constantly wearing out and dying off, and need to be replaced. For example, the red cells in our blood, which carry oxygen and give our blood its colour, have a lifespan of just 120 days, so every four months we will have completely replaced our red blood cells, producing billions of new cells. The numbers involved are unimaginably huge, but our bodies get them exactly right. If they made too few new red blood cells we would soon become anaemic, pale, tired and breathless, whereas if too many cells were made we would develop a disease called polycythaemia, which leads to things like blood clots, abnormal bleeding and strokes. Throughout our lives, from the moment of conception to the second we die, the process of cell division, cell growth, goes on, and is precisely controlled to make sure we have exactly the number of cells we need.

Cell growth is controlled by our genes. These are the microscopic chemical packages we inherit from our parents that determine what we are and who we are. Our genes tell our cells when to divide, when to reproduce. Every cell in our bodies carries a copy of our genes, so every one of our cells has this built-in command system to control everything it does, and to make sure it gets it right.

A cancer begins when a gene becomes damaged or faulty and starts to give the wrong instructions to a cell, telling it to multiply when it shouldn't.

In the 1960s an American scientist called Howard Springer did an experiment where he injected just a single cancer cell into a laboratory mouse. A few weeks later the mouse died of the cancer. This experiment showed that a life-threatening cancer could begin with changes in just a single cell.

So if just one of the genes which control cell division, in just one of the countless millions of cells in our bodies, becomes faulty or, to use the scientific jargon, if it has undergone a mutation, then this single cell could cause a cancer to develop.

With so many cells making up our bodies the likelihood is that these mutations are happening all the time, but usually our immune system, our built-in natural defences, will recognize the rogue cell and destroy it before it can do any damage. But once every so often, for some reason, a cell will get under the radar of our immune system and start the cancer growing.

Timescales

People often think of cancers growing very fast, but the time from when a cell first becomes cancerous to the time that cancer begins to cause problems, or symptoms, is usually a matter of years. That single cell has to divide into two, the two into four, the four into eight, and so on. Each of these divisions doubles the number of cancer cells. Laboratory experiments suggest most cancer cells divide every few weeks or months.

However skilful your doctors, whatever amazing blood tests, scans and x-rays they have at their command, there is no way they can detect a single cancerous cell in the body. It is just too small to show up. About the earliest most cancers can be diagnosed is when they have reached a size of half a centimetre across (and the great majority of cancers are only discovered when they are considerably bigger than this).

By the time a cancer is half a centimetre in diameter it will contain more than a thousand million cells. The single cell that started the whole problem will have doubled more than 20 times to reach this number. And each of those doublings takes several weeks or months. Furthermore, as a cancer grows, the number of cells which are actually dividing, which are actually multiplying, reduces. This is because the cancer, which is an abnormal growth, can't get enough oxygen and nutrients from the blood to allow all of its cells to divide, so many of the cells have to have a rest. And as the cancer gets bigger the number of resting cells increases and the number of dividing cells gets smaller. So the rate of growth of the cancer slows as it gets older.

Putting all these numbers and facts together, this means that most cancers will have started years before they actually cause any symptoms. So for most of its life a cancer is completely invisible and undetectable.

The diversity of types of cancer

When that fertilized egg cell that we all grow from begins to divide, as the new cells multiply they also begin to specialize, taking on new identities to form all the different tissues and organs that make up our bodies. Some cells will become liver cells, some will become brain cells, some will become muscle cells, and so on. Just as the number of our cells increases so does their diversity, forming the literally hundreds of different cell types that are needed to make a healthy person.

As life progresses, cancerous changes can happen in almost any of these different cells. This means that there are several hundred different types of cancer that we can develop. And

Table 1   Common cancers: the approximate number of new cancers diagnosed each year in the UK

Cancer	Men	Women	Total
Breast	600	44,000	44,600
Lung	22,000	14,000	36,000
Bowel	19,000	16,000	35,000
Prostate	30,000	—	30,000
Bladder	9,000	3,500	12,500
Lymphoma	6,000	5,000	11,000
Stomach	6,500	3,500	10,000
Oesophagus	4,500	3,000	7,500
Melanoma	3,000	4,000	7,000
Ovary	—	7,000	7,000
Pancreas	3,000	3,500	6,500
Uterus	—	6,000	6,000
Kidney	3,500	2,000	5,500
Brain	2,500	2,000	4,500
Cervix	—	3,500	3,500

these different cancers will behave in different ways and need different treatments. So a cell in the breast that becomes cancerous, and years later grows to form a breast cancer, will produce a cancer that is very different from a bone cancer or a prostate cancer.

Some cancers, like breast, lung, bowel and prostate cancer, are very common, while others are extremely rare, with only a handful of new cases being discovered in the UK each year. Table 1 gives an idea of some of the numbers.

Each year there are also more than 70,000 non-melanoma skin cancers diagnosed. These are often missed off official statistics as they often behave more like benign tumours and are usually very curable.

Even when we look at the cancers that develop in a particular organ or tissue, they are not all the same. Just to give a couple of examples: the current World Health Organization classification of lung cancer lists over 60 different forms of the disease; non-Hodgkin's lymphoma is a type of cancer that affects lymph glands and lymph tissue, but there are more than 20 different types of non-Hodgkin's lymphoma, each of which has its own pattern of behaviour. Even cancers of the same type don't all behave the same way: some will grow more rapidly than others, some will spread to other parts of the body later than others, some will respond to one type of treatment, others to another.

An important point about all this variety is that you cannot use other people's experience to predict what will happen to you. If you have a friend or relative with a cancer of the stomach and you are diagnosed with a cancer of the womb, then your symptoms, the way your cancer is treated and the chances of long-term success from that treatment will be quite different. You simply can't compare the two – it's like saying that if you are going to go on holiday to Spain you know what it will be like because your friend went on holiday to North Wales and told you all about it. Your friend's experience will be very different from yours (you might even get better weather!). Even when two people have the same type of cancer, for example two women with breast cancer or two men with prostate cancer, the likelihood is that the details of their treatment will be different, they will have different side effects from those treatments, and the tests and check-ups they have after their treatment is over won't be the same. This isn't because one person's doctors know what they're doing and the other person's don't – it's because, just as each of us is a unique individual, so every cancer is slightly different. There may be some broad similarities, but when it comes to the fine detail no two people and no two cancers are exactly the same.

What are my chances?

These variations in the behaviour of cancers mean that some cancers are much more serious than others. At one extreme is the commonest of all skin cancers, a condition called a basal cell carcinoma, or rodent ulcer. Although these are cancers, they grow very slowly, they very rarely spread anywhere else, they are usually found at a very early stage when they are still only a few millimetres in size, and treatment is either a minor operation or a shot of radiotherapy, both of which can be given as an outpatient and both of which almost always lead to a cure. By contrast, a cancer growing in the pancreas, deep in the belly, often causes very few symptoms until it has reached a very advanced stage, when it is difficult to treat and so has a far lower chance of being completely cured. The message here is that the chances of successful treatment vary from person to person and cancer to cancer. The old belief that having cancer was a universal death sentence could not be more wrong. The latest statistics show that more than half of all people in the UK who get cancer will be cured – permanently and completely cured. Of the remainder, many will have years of good-quality, active, essentially normal life before their illness catches up with them.

The fact that every cancer is slightly different also means that it is impossible to predict exactly how each one will behave. Statistics give doctors a good idea of what to expect, but they don't give them the power of absolute prediction. So if you go to your specialist with a small basal cell carcinoma on the skin of your cheek, he or she will be able to tell you that there is a 99 per cent chance of a cure, but what the specialist won't be able to tell you is whether or not you are the one person in 100 where the cancer will come back and need more treatment. Your specialist can give you the odds, but not the result of the race.

Benign or malignant?

Let's break off at this point to talk about the words that are used to describe cancer. We have said that a cancer develops when cell growth gets out of control. But there are two types of abnormal cell growth: benign and malignant. Both of these lead to tumours being formed, so a tumour may be either benign or malignant. A cancer is a malignant cell growth. A benign growth, a benign tumour, is not a cancer. A malignant growth, a malignant tumour, is a cancer. So if you are told you have a brain tumour, or a growth in your brain, it doesn't necessarily mean you have a cancer – the condition could be completely benign. It is only if you are told you have a malignant tumour, or a malignant growth, that you know you have a cancer.

There are two key differences between a benign growth and a malignant growth. As a benign tumour grows, it pushes aside the organs and tissues around it – it elbows them out of the way. As a malignant tumour – a cancer – grows, it eats into and destroys the organs and tissues that surround it. Benign growths may cause symptoms or problems by pressing on nearby tissues and organs, but cancers cause more damage because they actually erode those same tissues and organs. This means that when someone has an operation to remove a benign growth the surgery is usually fairly simple, since the tumour can easily be separated from, shelled out from, the tissues that surround it. With a cancer, the only way it can be removed completely is by taking a margin of normal tissue from around the growth, to make sure that all those microscopic strands of cancer cells invading, eating into their neighbouring structures, have been cut out, along with the central core of the growth.

The other difference is that cancers can spread to other places. Most cancers start in one place, in one organ. This is called the primary cancer. As that cancer grows, cells will break off from it and travel in the blood stream, or through the lymph vessels, to other parts of the body. Some of those cells will lodge in other organs and begin to multiply to form secondary cancers. Another word for these secondary cancers is metastases. So, for example, as a bowel cancer grows, if it is not treated then with time it will send off cells into the blood stream that will go to the liver, and sometimes also the lungs, and these will form secondary bowel cancers in those organs – liver and lung metastases from the primary bowel cancer. By contrast, a benign bowel tumour will never send off seedlings of cells, will never form secondaries or metastases. This is true however large the benign tumour is. Being benign or malignant has nothing to do with size – some of the largest tumours that occur in the human body are completely benign.

A final point to mention is that when a cancer spreads, when it forms metastases, those secondary cancers behave like the primary cancer. So if a prostate cancer spreads to the bones, then the secondary growth in the bone is made up of prostate cancer cells, not bone cancer cells, and will behave in a different way and need very different treatments from a cancer that starts in the bone – a primary bone cancer. This is something that the media often get confused over. Newspaper reports frequently have stories about famous people who have developed 'liver cancer'. In fact, primary liver cancers, malignant growths starting in the liver, are quite rare, but secondary cancers in the liver from primary cancers in the bowel or the breast or the lungs are very common. What those newspaper stories should say, if they are going to be accurate, is that the celebrity has a secondary liver cancer, or cancer that has spread to the liver from somewhere else in his or her body – but that is probably too technical for most journalists!

Back to the beginning: genes

In one way we can look at cancer as being a very natural process. With the infinite number of cell divisions that take place in our bodies from the moment we are conceived to the moment we die, it is hardly surprising that once in a while something goes wrong with the system, and a cell, or a handful of cells, somewhere, some time, slips out of control and declares independence, growing in its own way at its own speed, forming a new colony that goes on, often many years later, to appear as a potentially lethal cancer. Given the number of cell divisions that go on during our lifetimes, the wonder is that it doesn't happen more often.

When that process of cell division does slip out of control it is because something has gone wrong with one of our genes, causing it to malfunction and to send out the wrong signals, triggering the beginning of a cancer. Although scientists and doctors now believe this is the way all cancers start, we only know of a limited number of genes that can actually lead to a cancer developing when they are damaged or mutate. For example, in breast cancer there are two genes, called BRCA1 and BRCA2. If either of these is faulty then the chances of the person who has that gene developing a breast cancer some time during her (or his) life are far higher than for people whose genes are normal. But only one in 20 people who get breast cancer have abnormal BRCA1 or BRCA2 genes. So, most breast cancers must be due to other gene mutations which have yet to be discovered. Looking for the genes that cause cancer is one of the most active areas in medical research today, and more are being discovered all the time.

Having an abnormal cancer gene does not mean that you will definitely get a particular type of cancer, but it does increase your risk and means that you are more likely to develop that cancer than someone who does not have the gene. The degree of risk varies from gene to gene. This means that some people who have one of these genes may never get that cancer, though most probably will. It also means that many people who don't have the gene will still get that cancer because they develop a mutation in another gene.

How do you get a faulty gene?

Faulty genes can be either inherited or acquired.

Inherited faulty genes are passed down from one genera-tion to the next. They are passed on by a mother or father in the single egg or sperm that came together at the moment of conception. As the cells multiply, these abnormal genes are reproduced. They are there before birth, and there is nothing that can be done to avoid them. There is much more informa-tion about inherited cancer genes in the next chapter.

Acquired faulty genes are genes which undergo a mutation some time during your life. The exact causes of these muta-tions, the precise biochemical mechanisms which bring them about, largely remain a mystery. But there are a lot of things that we know make these mutations more likely and increase the chances of a cancer developing. These include our environ-ment, the world around us, the choices that we make in the way we lead our lives, and some other illnesses, in particular certain types of infection. In later chapters we will look at these different factors and what can be done to reduce their chances of causing cancer – how you can reduce your risk.

3

Cancers that can be inherited

Introduction

There is quite a lot of publicity these days about inherited cancer: cancers caused by faulty genes passed down through families from one generation to another. In fact, these make up only a tiny minority of all cancers. Among the most commonly occurring cancers, about one in 20 breast cancers and one in 25 bowel cancers are due to inheriting faulty genes. But because people are more aware of this risk there is often a lot of unnecessary worry – anxiety that if a relative gets cancer it might mean that you are going to get it too.

Just how common that belief is was highlighted in a survey carried out by the charity Cancerbackup with Genes Reunited early in 2007. Out of 1,000 people questioned, an amazing 91 per cent falsely believed that if someone in their family had cancer, they would have a greater than average chance of getting cancer themselves, and six out of ten thought that a history of cancer in the family was the biggest risk factor for getting the disease (actually, the biggest single risk factor is age: the older you are, the longer you live, the more likely it is that you will get cancer). In reality, for most types of cancer, the fact that a close relative has had the disease won't increase your risk at all.

Cancer is very common: as many as one in three of us will get it at some time during our lives. This means that in any family someone is likely to get cancer. So how can you tell if this is because there is a faulty gene being carried by one or more of your relatives, or due to something else? Gene testing is one obvious option, but this is a complex, very time-consuming process: it can take many months to get answers, and even then those answers are not always reliable. The simplest and clearest way of getting an idea of whether or not a faulty gene is involved is to look at the pattern of cancer within a family. This involves tracing the medical history of all your close relatives, finding out which of them developed cancer, the type of cancer they had, and the age at which their cancer was discovered. Once you have this information you can get a pretty good idea of whether or not there is a genetic risk.

Before we look at a couple of examples with breast and bowel cancer, there are two phrases that need to be explained. When doctors are trying to work out whether or not a faulty gene is the cause of a cancer, they look at the medical history of the person's 'first-degree' and 'second-degree' relatives. A first-degree relative is a parent, a brother or sister, or a child of that person. They must also be blood relatives, so if they are adopted then the medical history of their adopted mother and father doesn't count, although the medical history of their children would. A second-degree relative is a grandparent, grandchild, aunt, uncle, niece, nephew, half-sister or half-brother.

Breast cancer

By looking at the medical history of her first- and second-degree relatives, the National Institute of Health and Clinical Excellence (NICE) has worked out a schedule for predicting a woman's risk of developing breast cancer as a result of a faulty gene.

The NICE schedule looks at three levels of risk:

- Normal population risk: at this level, out of every 100 women, 17 or fewer would be expected to develop breast cancer at some time during their lives.
- Raised risk: in this group, out of every 100 women, somewhere between 17 and 30 would develop breast cancer.

- High risk: in this group more than 30 out of every 100 women would develop breast cancer.

NICE says that a woman falls into the raised risk group if she has one of the following in her family:

- one first-degree relative who was diagnosed with breast cancer before the age of 40;
- one first-degree relative and one second-degree relative diagnosed after an average age of 50;
- two first-degree relatives diagnosed with breast cancer after an average age of 50.

A woman would fall into NICE's high risk group if she had any of the following in her family:

- one first-degree relative and one second-degree relative diagnosed with breast cancer before an average age of 50;
- two first-degree relatives diagnosed with breast cancer before an average age of 50;
- three or more first- or second-degree relatives diagnosed with breast cancer at any age;
- one first-degree relative who developed cancer in both her breasts, with one of those cancers being diagnosed before she was 50;
- one first-degree male relative who developed breast cancer at any age;
- one first-degree or second-degree relative with ovarian cancer at any age *and* one first- or second-degree relative with breast cancer at any age (one of the two should be a first-degree relative).

Even among those women who fall into NICE's raised or high risk group, only a minority will actually be carriers of one of the faulty genes BRCA1 and BRCA2 which, as we saw in the previous chapter, have been linked to breast cancer. The underlying reason for the increased risk among the majority remains a mystery – there may well be other faulty genes that have still to be discovered, or there may be some other factor that is as yet unknown.

Using these NICE guidelines, very few women will find that they have an increased risk of getting breast cancer because of their family history. For most women the chance of inheriting a gene, or a tendency, to develop breast cancer is small. The fact that one or more relatives may have had another type of cancer, or even that someone has had breast cancer, doesn't mean you are more at risk, unless the person with breast cancer was a close relative who had her cancer at a young age (under 40).

For those women who do find they are at more than average risk, the first thing to do is to see their family doctor, who will go through the family medical history and should be able to confirm whether or not there is a greater risk and, if there is, whether or not they need to see a specialist. If that specialist then confirms that there is an increased risk, there are a number of ways of dealing with this. Depending on the level of risk and the wishes of the individual woman, this might just mean regular self-examination of her breasts (looking for any lumps, changes in the shape of the breast or changes in the shape of the nipples, or any bleeding or discharge from the nipples) and regular breast screening (which for women over 50 will involve having a mammogram, a breast x-ray, and in younger women will mean having a special type of scan called an MRI scan – this is because younger women have denser, firmer breast tissue which makes mammograms less accurate at picking up cancers). If the risk is greater then other options include hormonal therapy (see p. 86) or even surgery to remove both breasts. This is called a prophylactic bilateral mastectomy and sounds a drastic choice, but the evidence is that those women who decide to go for it, having weighed up their risks and been carefully counselled before making their decision, usually cope with the operation very well and go on to enjoy a good quality of life with greatly reduced anxiety.

Bowel cancer

Bowel cancer affects about one in 50 people in the UK at some time during their lives. About one in every 25 of these cancers will be due to a faulty gene passed down through the family.

The link between the number of family members who have had bowel cancer, or other cancers, and the exact risk of someone getting a bowel cancer is even more complicated than that for breast cancer. But the all-important sign that a bowel cancer may be caused by a faulty gene is the age of the person when that cancer is first discovered. Bowel cancer generally affects people in late middle age or old age; the average time of diagnosis in the UK is around the age of 70. By contrast, those cancers which are linked to an inherited gene usually appear before the age of 45. So people who have a first-degree relative who develops a bowel cancer over the age of 45 may be at slightly increased risk of getting the disease themselves but do not need special tests or screening (although they should always see their doctor promptly if they develop any bowel problems, especially any bleeding from the back passage, and they should, of course, take up the invitation to join the national bowel cancer screening programme when they are 60 or over). But if someone has a first-degree relative who develops a bowel cancer before the age of 45, or has two first-degree relatives who have developed a cancer of their colon or rectum at any age, then that person's risk is increased to three or four times that of the rest of the population and he or she should get the advice of the GP. This will almost always mean referral to a specialist for further assessments.

When bowel cancer is due to a faulty gene, this is the result of one of two different conditions. The first of these is called familial adenomatous polyposis (FAP) and is caused by a mutation on a gene known as the APC gene. This leads to the development of thousands of benign tumours, or polyps, in the bowel. Inevitably, with time, one or more of these will become a cancer, and there is virtually a 100 per cent risk of developing a colon cancer. In this situation, the first-degree relatives of the person who has developed the cancer should be offered genetic counselling, and should be tested to see if they too have the gene. If they are found to have an abnormal APC gene, they will be offered a screening test every year, and if polyps begin to appear they may be advised to have surgery to remove part of their bowel in order to prevent a cancer appearing.

The other condition is called hereditary non-polyposis colorectal cancer syndrome (HNPCC) or the Lynch syndrome. Here the damaged gene does not cause any polyps to be formed, but does lead to about a seven in ten chance of getting a bowel cancer at some time during life. The likelihood that someone might have an abnormal HNPCC gene is once again based on the family's medical history, using a set of guidelines known as the Modified Amsterdam Criteria. If these suggest that the person may be at risk, genetic counselling and testing will be offered. If the test shows the presence of the gene, then a screening test looking at the bowel (called a colonoscopy) is likely to be offered and to be repeated every few years, so that if a cancer does develop it will be found at an early stage when it is still treatable and highly curable.

Overall, only about one in every 2,500 people is a carrier of either the FAP or HNPCC gene mutation, but, as with breast cancer, bowel cancer does appear to be more common in some families even when an obvious faulty gene cannot be found. If you have a close relative or relatives who have been affected by bowel cancer, the best thing to do is to have a chat with your GP so he or she can consider your family's medical history and work out whether you really do have an increased risk or not. If together you do discover you are more likely than other people to get bowel cancer, your GP will be able to arrange specialist advice to work out your real risk and advise about genetic testing, screening or other measures that may need to be taken to help reduce your risk.

Other cancers

There are a number of other cancers where it is well recognized that a history of that particular cancer among close relatives can increase your chance of getting the disease, although in most cases either the precise faulty genes that might be to blame have not been identified, or the exact risks have not been worked out quite so clearly as in breast cancer and bowel cancer. These include prostate cancer, cancer of the womb, cancer of the ovary, stomach cancer and cancer of the pancreas. There are also some links between the different cancer types: if two close relatives are diagnosed with one having breast cancer and the other a cancer of the ovary, then this makes a faulty gene more likely to be the cause of their illness. Similarly, having bowel cancer and cancer of the womb in two close relatives suggests a faulty gene as the cause.

All this goes to show that we are still at a fairly early stage in working out the genes that may give rise to different types of cancer when they are damaged or undergo a mutation. New cancer genes are being discovered all the time, and the relationship between the genes we already know about and their involvement in the formation of different types of cancer is also a rapidly expanding area of research. At the present time, however, the evidence is still that most cancers are not caused by inheriting a faulty gene from our parents. This means that, for the great majority of people, if one of your close relatives gets cancer there is no need to worry that this makes you more at risk. However, if one or more of your nearest and dearest have had cancer, or have recently been diagnosed with the disease, and you are worried, the thing to do is to go and have a talk with your GP and get advice as to whether or not you really are more likely to get cancer or not. If your GP does feel there is any increased risk, he or she will either be able to advise you what to do or will arrange for you to see a specialist, who can put you fully in the picture and explain the various ways in which your risk can be reduced.

4

Lifestyle and cancer risk

Introduction

Experts differ in their estimates, suggesting that anywhere from a quarter to three-quarters of all cancers are the result of things in our own lifestyle, things that we can control and are responsible for. These include whether or not we smoke, what we eat and drink, our weight and our levels of physical activity, and, if you are a woman, whether or not you use the contraceptive pill or HRT. There is also the issue of how much we expose ourselves to the sun – which we will look at in the next chapter.

Smoking: the root of the problem

Smoking causes cancer. The biggest cancer risk from cigarette smoking is lung cancer. When you breathe cigarette smoke you are taking in three things: tar, carbon monoxide and nicotine.

Tar is the real cancer risk. It is made up of hundreds of different chemicals, many of which are known to cause cancer. Most of the tar that a smoker breathes in gets trapped and stays in the lungs, where the chemicals do their deadly work on the cells lining the airways, causing the gene mutations that, over the years, will lead to potentially fatal bronchogenic carcinomas: lung cancers.

Carbon monoxide is a poisonous gas. It is the lethal ingredient in the fumes of faulty boilers and gas fires that sometimes kill people. Those people die from asphyxiation, suffocation; and in the tiny doses that are found in cigarette smoke the carbon monoxide slowly poisons the lungs, leading to chronic breathing problems: bronchitis and emphysema.

Nicotine is the chemical that makes smokers smoke. It is very highly addictive. One reason for this is that it reaches the brain within a matter of seconds of taking a puff, and so it is an instant stimulus. Apart from being addictive, nicotine itself doesn't do any real harm. The problem with cigarettes is that, in order to get the nicotine, you can't avoid the cancer-causing tar and the lung-damaging carbon monoxide. The pleasure of the nicotine fix comes at the cost of breathing in the carcinogenic cocktail of chemicals in the tar and the poisonous carbon monoxide.

Over the years I worked with three doctors who were heavy smokers (more than 20 cigarettes a day). They are all now dead: two died from lung cancer and one from carcinoma of the pancreas, another smoking-related cancer. They all knew the risk they were taking, they all chose to take that risk, and they all paid the price of their decision.

How big is the problem?

Each year in the UK more than 20,000 men and 13,000 women die from lung cancer. In other words, on average someone dies from lung cancer every 15 minutes. More than nine out of every ten of these fatal cancers will have been caused by smoking. Although it is the biggest killer, lung cancer isn't the only problem. Smoking increases the risk of getting a whole range of other cancers, including bladder cancer, cancers of the mouth and throat, cancer of the pancreas and cancer of the cervix. And, of course, there are the other smoking-related diseases: chronic bronchitis, emphysema and heart disease, all of which can be fatal. The bottom line of these medical hazards is that one out of every two people who smoke more than 20 cigarettes a day will die from a smoking-related disease.

The risk of getting lung cancer increases directly with the number of cigarettes you smoke each day. The more you smoke, the greater your chance of getting the disease. Smoke ten a day and you are ten times more likely than a non-smoker to end up with lung cancer; smoke 20 a day and you are 20 times more likely. The youngest person I ever met among my patients with lung cancer was in his mid-thirties. He worked as a barman and somehow managed to smoke 120 cigarettes a day (how he found both the time and the money, I never understood). Sadly, despite an initial dramatic improvement with chemotherapy, he rapidly relapsed and died within three months of the time I first saw him. Lung cancer kills, and unfortunately, despite the many advances in treatment of cancer overall, it remains one of the most resistant to cure; in the UK the chances of surviving five years after a diagnosis of carcinoma of the bronchus is only about one in 20. Over the last 35 years, while the overall cure rate for cancer has doubled, the figure for lung cancer has remained stubbornly unchanged. Prevention is better than cure, not only because the cure is not particularly pleasant, but because the chances of achieving it are pretty remote.

The close link between cigarette smoking and lung cancer is something most people know, and about two out of every three smokers say they would like to give up because of the health hazards. But despite this, about one in four people (26 per cent of all men and 23 per cent of all women) keep up the habit, and these numbers haven't changed over the last five years: as a nation we are not smoking less. Simply being aware of the possible hellfire of lung cancer, or other lethal illnesses, isn't enough to stop people, and the reason for this is that smoking is an addiction. Nicotine, as mentioned earlier, is a powerful addictive drug, and giving up is not easy. Knowing the health risks they are running, and having this message backed up by leaflets and booklets, and even one-to-one talks with their family doctor, only helps about one person in 20 who want to stop smoking to achieve their ambition. Most people need more help. And 'help' is the key word. Simply preaching that smoking is bad for you isn't going to be enough to make most smokers quit.

Incidentally, the recently introduced smoking ban in public places in the UK has been brought in with the aim of reducing illness, including lung cancer. But there is a time lag between smoking and the development of lung cancer: it takes 20 years or more for the disease to develop. This means that if the ban is effective it will be decades before we see the results in terms of fewer people getting carcinoma of the bronchus. Also, the immediate evidence as to whether the ban is doing what is hoped is debatable. In Scotland, the first part of the UK to introduce the ban, figures show that since its introduction in March 2006 the number of packets of cigarettes bought each week has gone up by over 60,000. All this is not to say that the ban is not a good thing – as a non-smoker and an oncologist I definitely approve – but it is not going to achieve the health benefits it aspires to overnight.

The benefits of not smoking

As nearly everybody knows, the best way to reduce your risk of getting lung cancer is not to smoke, and never to have smoked in the past. There are a few cases caused by passive smoking and non smoking-related causes, but overall a lifelong non-smoker would be very unlucky indeed to get lung cancer. So, if you don't smoke and never have done, that's great, and your chances of getting any one of a whole range of different cancers are far less than those of a smoker.

What if you were a smoker and have recently managed to give up? First, congratulations on a great achievement. And yes, your risk of getting lung cancer will reduce. Overall, your chances of getting a lung cancer will have halved after ten years of not smoking. And the longer you stop smoking, the lower your risk. Overall, the likelihood of getting lung cancer is reduced by more than 80 per cent for non-smokers compared to those who carry on smoking heavily (more than 20 ciga-rettes a day). There is also an age factor. The longer you smoke, the higher your risk of getting lung cancer, so the younger you stop the more quickly your risk reduces. Put another way, if someone stops smoking before the age of 35, then he or she will have the same life-expectancy as a non-smoker. But even if you are in your fifties and have been a lifelong smoker, stopping can more than halve your chance of getting a lung cancer.

One final set of figures to encourage any of you who are smokers to give up: on average, people who stop when they are 30 have an extra ten years of life compared to those who carry on smoking, and even if they only stop when they're 60 they still get an extra three years. It is never too late to stop.

What about 'half-measures'? Suppose you cut back, or change to a pipe or cigars? There is some evidence that reducing the number of cigarettes you smoke each day helps a bit, but only a bit. The figures are that if you followed 100 lifelong smokers of 20 a day, then, by the age of 75, 50 of them would have devel-oped lung cancer; by reducing to ten cigarettes or fewer each day, the number of cancers would reduce to about 37. You've slightly reduced the odds, but there's still a better than one in three chance that you'll end up with lung cancer. Changing to a pipe or cigars is a slightly more effective way of reducing your risk: you will be about 50 per cent less likely to develop lung cancer than a heavy smoker. But that is still almost 50 per cent more than a non-smoker. Cutting back or changing to cigars or a pipe is a half-measure, or even less than a half-measure; if you can, it is far better to give up completely.

Giving up

If you are a smoker, the one thing you can do that will lower your chance of getting cancer is … stop. Quit. Give up. That, of course, is easier said than done.

The key to success is motivation, actually wanting to stop. While writing this chapter I took a break and went to the National Theatre to listen to an interview with a famous playwright. He recounted how, the last time he had been there to see a play, he had gone out on to the terrace in the interval to enjoy one of his many cigarettes of the day. The next thing he remembered was waking up in an ambulance on the way to St Thomas's Hospital, having collapsed.

'So did you give up smoking?' asked the interviewer.

'No,' replied the playwright, 'I gave up going to the theatre.'

Despite an even more obvious health warning than the message on his cigarette packets, he was clearly not motivated to quit. But surveys suggest that almost three out of four smokers would like to quit, and more than half say they intend to do so in the next 12 months.

The stronger the desire, the greater the chance of success. Most of those who say they would like to give up cite fears about their health as their main reason, and very rightly so. But another aspect is the sheer cost of smoking. Given the number of cigarettes you have to smoke to get it, lung cancer is an expensive disease – you need to spend about £10,000. Back in the 1950s, my father was never seen without his pipe and my mother always had a cigarette close to hand. But then came a huge cultural change – we got our first television. Money was scarce, and the only way the new TV could be afforded was by hire purchase. The only way the repayments could be met was by my father giving up smoking, which he did. Each week the money that he would have spent on tobacco went into – appropriately – an empty tobacco tin, and was ready to pay off the instalments at the end of each month. When the 'never-never' debt was finally cleared, we owned our own TV and my father was a non-smoker, and he stayed that way.

If you do want to stop, you are probably going to need help. Research suggests that using willpower alone, only about one in 30 smokers who want to stop actually will. The two main approaches to backing up personal motivation, supporting your desire to stop, are counselling and medication.

Counselling, or intensive behavioural support, has been shown to work; about one in ten smokers who go through a course will manage to give up the habit. The courses are run by specially trained smoking cessation counsellors. There are a variety of different ways in which the counselling is done, and no one approach seems better than any other. Also, whether you have the sessions on a one-to-one basis or in a group doesn't seem to make any difference to the chances of success. In the UK, counselling services to help people give up smoking are now available on the NHS, and your family doctor ought to be able to arrange this for you.

Medication to help people give up smoking comes in two main types: nicotine replacement therapy and drugs called Zyban (buproprion) and Champix (verenicline). As with counselling, about one in ten smokers who want to give up and use nicotine replacement therapy to help them find that they succeed.

Nicotine replacement therapy comes in a number of forms: you can chew it as a gum, stick it on your skin as a transdermal patch, suck it as a lozenge, squirt it up your nose as a nasal spray, take it as a tablet which you put under your tongue and let dissolve, or inhale it from a puffer (like those used by people with asthma). All these different preparations work in the same way: they release nicotine into your blood stream. That release occurs more slowly than with cigarette smoking so there isn't the same instant fix, which is why the replacement therapy isn't a complete substitute for smoking for some people. But it will still calm the nicotine receptors in the brain and will greatly reduce the addictive craving for a cigarette. Also, since none of the types of nicotine replacement contain either tar or carbon monoxide, they are much safer than cigarettes – in fact, there appear to be no serious harmful long-term effects from their use. All forms of nicotine replacement therapy are now available on prescription on the NHS or, if you prefer, the patches, gum and lozenges can all be bought over the counter at pharmacists or supermarkets.

Zyban is a drug that was originally developed as an anti-depressant. When it was being tested in clinical trials it was also found to reduce people's need to smoke. The exact chemical mechanism behind this remains uncertain, but there is no doubt that for many smokers it will reduce their craving for a cigarette. It is taken as a slow-release tablet, once a day. Very rarely it can cause seizures, so it is not recommended for people with a history of epilepsy, but other side effects, if they occur, are usually mild, a dry mouth, insomnia or a skin rash being the commonest. Zyban is available on prescription on the NHS in the UK. Recently, another tablet, Champix, has also been approved in the UK. Studies show this is as effective, or even more effective, than Zyban. It works by stopping nicotine reaching receptors in the brain, and so reduces the craving for cigarettes; if you do succumb and have a puff, this makes it less rewarding than it would have been because you don't get the nicotine fix. Champix is taken once or twice a day and, like Zyban, is available on prescription.

Counselling and medication can be used together, and studies suggest that combining them does help, with as many as one in five smokers being able to give up as a result.

If you are thinking of giving up (and please do), the NHS is keen to help and strongly supports smokers who want to stop: it spent more than £50 million on its Stop Smoking Services in 2006. A first step would be to see your family doctor, who can give you advice about planning your campaign, put you in touch with counselling services and arrange prescriptions for medications if you need them. Or you could phone the NHS smoking helpline on 0800 169 0 169. Do give it a try. You would be doing yourself a favour, with a real chance of improving your health, drastically reducing your chances of getting cancer and saving a large amount of money.

Pan

Cigarette smoking is the strongest link between tobacco and cancer, but another hazard is the combination of tobacco and pan. Pan (or paan) has been part of the culture of people in parts of the Indian subcontinent and Far East for thousands of years. The main ingredient of pan is the areca nut, which is dried, shredded and mixed with slaked lime. This mixture is then rolled in a leaf from the Piper betel vine, to form a betel quid. Tobacco is frequently added to the mixture, and sometimes other ingredients as well (including spices such as cardamom, coconut and saffron). Another variation is the addition of Zarda, which is boiled tobacco. In the UK pan is also available as Paan masala, a readymade packet that may contain either the whole mixture or just the spices. Paan is often combined with tobacco, and this increases the cancer risk even more.

Once it has been prepared, the quid is placed in the mouth between the teeth and the lining of the cheek, releasing various chemicals into the blood stream. These chemicals have a number of effects, including a feeling of well-being (the use of the slaked lime helps speed the release of these chemicals, thus giving a rapid 'lift').

Using pan occasionally may not be harmful, but with regular use people do become dependent on, or even addicted to, the mixture. The degree of dependence is thought to be about the same as to cocaine, so it is a strong compulsion. People are more likely to become dependent if tobacco is included in the pan.

There is now definite evidence that people who use pan frequently have an increased likelihood of getting cancer of the lining of the mouth. The risk of a regular pan user getting a mouth cancer is between two and four times greater than for a non-user. This risk seems to increase with the number of pan taken and the length of time the person has been a user. Pan can also increase the risk of other cancers, including cancer of the throat and oesophagus (gullet). There is also recent evidence that it may be linked to the development of liver cancer as well.

There has been debate as to whether the harmful effects of pan are due to the addition of tobacco to the mixture; evidence is that use of the areca nut on its own still carries a risk of causing cancer, but that this risk is increased by adding tobacco to the mixture.

Diet

There is probably more written about what we eat and how it relates to cancer than about any other possible causes of the disease. Unfortunately a huge number of these reports are unreliable or irrelevant, or both. But they are enormously popular with the media, and any publication in a scientific journal that links something we eat or drink to cancer is bound to get its quota of column inches in one or more national newspapers. In the space of a few weeks during 2007, the British national daily papers carried stories about broccoli, cauliflower, chokeberries, black carrots, radishes, eating organic fruit rather than 'ordinary' fruit, eating more eggs when you are a teenager, strawberry cocktails, tea (two cups each day), purple grape juice and cloudy apple juice, all of which were said to reduce the risk of various cancers. There were also more confusing reports about multivitamins, grapefruit and coffee, where one study had said they helped prevent cancer and another had said they increased the cancer risk. Working out the truth about the relationship between our diet and our chance of getting cancer is not easy. A big part of the problem is the way we get the evidence.

How do they know?

Let us look again at where the evidence comes from. There are two main sources: studies on people and laboratory experiments.

There are two broad types of studies on people: retrospective and prospective. In a retrospective study, a group of people is asked to look back over the previous five, ten, 20 or whatever number of years and answer a range of questions about the diet followed by members of the group. The researcher then looks at the people in the group who have had cancer to see if there is any difference between their answers and those of the rest of the group. In a prospective study a group of volunteers is selected and observed for a period of years. These studies fall into two types. In one, the volunteers might be asked to keep a record of what they eat and see how this relates to whether or not they get cancer. In the other, it may be that half the group will have some form of intervention, for example taking a regular vitamin supplement or cutting red meat out of their diet, while the other half will carry on as normal. At the end of the study the numbers and types of cancers in both groups are compared to see if there is any difference.

Both methods have their limitations. Both rely on people recalling, or recording, their diet over a period of time – and not everybody can be relied on to be completely accurate, or completely honest. They also don't allow for other factors: for example, people who are very careful about their diet are likely to be generally more health conscious and look after themselves better than people who eat a very poor diet, so the fact that the careful people are less likely to get cancer may be due to other things they are doing rather than just a result of what they are, or are not, eating.

When it comes to laboratory experiments, the results are even more uncertain in terms of their relevance to human cancers. Quite reasonably, scientists are continually working to try and find chemicals that might either cause or protect against cancer.

A first step in doing this is to test those chemicals in the laboratory. The key words in that sentence are 'a first step' – even if studies with cultures of cells in Petri dishes or with unsuspecting mice look interesting, it will need repeated testing to confirm those findings, and then years of clinical investigation, with human studies, before their true worth is known. Over the decades countless thousands of chemicals have been identified in laboratory experiments that appear to either cause cancers or kill off cancer cells, but only a tiny handful of these have ever been shown to be linked to cancer in people, or to be of any use in its treatment.

To give just one example: in 2005, in the journal *Molecular Cancer Therapeutics*, researchers reported that the chemical pentameric procyanidin, which is one of the countless chemicals found in cocoa, stopped the growth of breast cancer cells being grown in culture dishes in their labs. The scientists were appropriately cautious about their findings, stressing the need for more work, and they issued a press statement saying that their study 'does not mean that people who eat chocolate will either reduce their cancer risks, or that eating chocolate will treat a current case'. Yet one of the UK's leading national newspapers reported their research with the headline 'Chocolate helps fight cancer' and began the article with 'Eating chocolate could help beat cancer, according to university researchers …'. This is by no means an isolated case – it happens all the time. As I have said before, all too often the media are interested in the story, not the science, and as a result we are constantly misled into believing that 'university researchers' or 'leading scientists' have shown that something we eat or drink or which makes up some other part of our everyday life, like hairsprays or deodorants, is either a sure route to getting cancer or a magic means of protecting against it. The message is 'reader, beware!': usually approach any of these stories armed with a large dose of salt.

A final point to mention is that because different methods are used for different studies, and because of the various sources of error inherent in those methods, different studies may give different answers to the same question. It is only by looking at the results of a number of different studies (after having excluded those that are completely unreliable) and balancing their findings and conclusions that some idea of an answer can be reached. For example, for many years it has been widely believed that eating a diet rich in vegetables and fruit helps protect against bowel cancer. The actual results from scientific studies were variable, some supporting this idea, others not. In 2007 the *Journal of the National Cancer Institute* published a major analysis of the data from 14 of the most important papers, looking at more than 750,000 people. This concluded that, overall, 'fruit and vegetable intakes were not strongly associated with colon cancer risk'. The message here is that you can't rely on the results of a single study in isolation to give you a clear answer: those results have to be backed up by consistent, similar findings from a number of other investigators.

So what about diet and cancer?

When you exclude all the laboratory testing studies and all those reports based on people trying to remember what they have eaten in the past, and focus on the most accurate type of research – large prospective studies following up populations of thousands of people over a period of time – there is surprisingly little evidence for a clear link between the things we eat and the risk of getting certain types of cancer.

Perhaps the strongest link is between eating red meat, and getting bowel cancer (and, to a lesser extent, prostate cancer). The suggestion that a meat-rich diet might be linked to bowel cancer first came from circumstantial evidence. Bowel cancer is much commoner in those countries with a high consumption of red meat, and people who move from countries where bowel cancer is less common to countries where it is more common tend to increase their risk. Similarly, between 1950 and 1990 meat consumption in Japan rose tenfold, and during the same time the rate of large bowel cancer increased to five times its previous level. Observations like these have led to formal scientific studies monitoring large populations of volunteers over a period of time. The pooled results of these reports suggest that eating an average of more than 100–20 grams of red meat each day increases your risk of bowel cancer by about 25 per cent, and eating more than 30 grams of processed red meat each day increases your risk by 30–50 per cent (processed red meat includes things like sausages, pâtés and pies). Based on these figures, while the overall chance of getting bowel cancer is that it will affect one person in 50, among people who eat large amounts of red meat regularly that figure falls to about one in 25 to one in 35; the odds have shortened, and the risk is increased. Although they are based on more than 50 different research studies, these results are still not absolutely conclusive, but they do strongly suggest there is a link between heavy consumption of red meat and a greater risk of getting bowel cancer. Other studies have suggested that a diet rich in red meat or processed red meat could also increase the risk of breast cancer and stomach cancer, but there are fewer reports about these cancers and the evidence-base is not as strong as that for bowel cancer, though this could change with time. However, these results do support the general message that too much red meat or too many red meat products may increase your cancer risk.

Another quite strong link, this time a positive one, is between lycopenes and a reduced risk of prostate cancer. Lycopene is a protein found in tomatoes, and it becomes even more concentrated when tomatoes are processed or cooked with oil. Lycopene is a potent anti-oxidant, and the general opinion is that anti-oxidants are a good thing when it comes to trying reduce our cancer risk. Certainly, studies looking prospectively at men's diets tend to support this view, since they suggest that a diet rich in tomatoes, or tomato products like purées and sauces, could reduce their chances of developing prostate cancer. Although the level of risk reduction varies considerably in different reports, all tend to show the same thing: a positive benefit.

It is important to mention that the likelihood of the things we eat increasing or reducing our risk of getting cancer depends not only on what we eat, and how much, but also how often we have them. Eating one steak won't give us bowel cancer, and eating two tomatoes won't stop us getting prostate cancer. We are talking about regular consumption or non-consumption of specific foods over a long period of time. This is another thing that often isn't made clear in media coverage of scientific reports on the subject; in many instances, especially with laboratory studies, the amounts of the food being studied that would have to be consumed on a regular basis in order to produce a harmful effect are far greater than most people would ever think of eating. What all this means is that a balanced diet is a safe diet, and it is best to avoid extremes.

Incidentally, researchers have found that, when it comes to diet and health, people would much rather take some sort of supplement to what they eat normally, than actually change what they eat. Understandably, this has led to a lot of research about the role of vitamin supplements in cancer prevention. The literature is vast, and the results of individual studies often give contradictory answers – some claiming to show great bene-fits, others showing no effect and others showing positive harm, with an actual increase in the number of cancers. The overall result is that there is no good evidence that taking regular vitamin supplements helps reduce the risk of getting cancer.

On balance

On balance, looking in detail at diet and trying to pick individual foods that will reduce the risk of cancer isn't terribly helpful. The best overall advice is to have plenty of fresh fruit and vegetables and to keep portions of red meat, especially processed meat, to two or three times a week. This will not only keep in line with what evidence there is for the risks and benefits of diet and cancer formation, but will fit in with the far stronger evidence for a healthy diet and the reduction in heart disease and diabetes.

While there are still many questions about what we eat and whether it may protect against cancer or increase our risk of getting it, there is little doubt that how much we eat is very important: the link between obesity and an increased risk of certain types of cancer is inescapable. But before looking at this, we should spend a moment considering drinking, as opposed to eating, and the question of alcohol and cancer.

Alcohol

The link between drinking alcohol and getting cancer is complicated. It is also something that the media regularly highlight, often in very alarmist ways, when any new scientific report on the subject appears. The evidence is that there are some cancers which are more likely to occur in moderate or heavy drinkers, and there are others where there is no evidence of such an increased risk.

It might help get an idea of who, from a medical point of view, is a moderate drinker and who is a heavy drinker. The UK government measures alcohol intake in units, with one unit being equal to eight grams of alcohol; this is roughly the same as a small (125 ml) glass of wine, or a pint of beer or a single measure of spirits. The official advice is that a woman should drink no more than 14 units each week and a man no more than 21. A moderate drinker is someone who drinks about this much; a heavy drinker would be someone who drinks a lot more.

The clearest evidence of a link between drinking alcohol and cancer comes from people with cancers of the throat (pharynx) and voice box (larynx). These cancers are also caused by smoking, and people who smoke and drink are much more likely to develop one of these cancers. So while a moderate drinker who is a non-smoker is slightly less than twice as likely as a non-drinker to get cancer of the pharynx or larynx, someone who is a heavy drinker (imbibing more than 40 units of alcohol each week) and a heavy smoker (smoking 30 or more cigarettes a day) is 35 times more likely than a teetotal non-smoker to get one or other of these cancers.

Cancers of the pharynx and larynx are not common and together make up only about 1 per cent of all cancers. Among the common cancers the two with most evidence of a link to alcohol are large bowel cancer and breast cancer, although in both of these the figures are much less dramatic than for the throat and voice box growths. In cancer of the large bowel (the colon or the rectum), moderate or heavy drinkers are about 10 per cent more likely than non-drinkers to get one of these tumours. What that figure means is that in the UK about 50 out of every 1,000 men and women will get a bowel cancer at some time during their lives. Among moderate and heavy drinkers that figure is likely to rise to about 55 out of every 1,000. So drinkers are at greater risk, but the odds are still very likely that they won't get the disease.

The link between alcohol and breast cancer is one that has attracted a lot of publicity in recent years. The widely quoted statistic is that for every glass of wine you drink each day (in other words, for every unit of alcohol you drink each day), you increase your risk of getting breast cancer by 6 per cent. What that actually means is that, overall, in every 1,000 women about 110 will develop breast cancer, the average age of onset being the late sixties. Among women who are moderate drinkers that figure would rise to about 117 out of every 1,000, and among heavy drinkers it may be as high as 130–40 out of every 1,000. Although this is still an increase, it is less frightening than the suggestion of some newspapers that every time you have a glass of wine your chances of getting breast cancer go up by 6 per cent – which would mean that once you had drunk two bottles of wine, you would be almost guaranteed to get breast cancer.

Other cancers where there is some evidence that regular drinking increases the risk include liver cancer and cancer of the gullet (cancer of the oesophagus). On the other hand, research has failed to show any link between alcohol and a number of other more common cancers, like prostate cancer and cancer of the ovary.

Why alcohol might increase someone's risk of getting cancer remains uncertain, although there are many theories. In general, though, the risks seem to depend on how much you drink, not what you drink: it is the alcohol intake that matters, not whether you have that as beer, wine or spirits. And it is also regular drinking that makes the difference – having a glass of sherry once a year at Christmas doesn't mean you will get cancer.

Statisticians have estimated that if everyone in the world stopped drinking alcohol, then cancer deaths would fall in men by about 5 per cent and in women by about 2 per cent. Some people think these are worrying numbers, and others think they are relatively unimportant. This reflects the fact that the whole subject of alcohol and health is very controversial. While there is no doubt that heavy drinking is harmful, there is good evidence that people who drink the equivalent of a glass of wine each day have a better life-expectancy than non-drinkers. When it comes to cancer, if you are a drinker who keeps close to the

Department of Health guidelines of 14 units for a woman or 21 for a man each week then you probably do have an increased risk, but that increased risk is pretty small. But if you want to make it even smaller, then being teetotal is one way of doing that.

Obesity: body weight and cancer

The evidence is overwhelming that being overweight increases our risk of getting cancer. Current estimates suggest that as many as one in five cancers in women, and slightly fewer in men, could be caused by being too heavy. Put another way, in the UK every year more than 10,000 new cancers are due to people not having a healthy body weight.

Being overweight is certainly not good for us. A large study in the USA has shown that men and women who are overweight live between three and seven years less than those with a normal weight. These figures are for non-smokers; if you are overweight and smoke, then the reduction in lifespan is anything up to 13 years.

Many of the health problems caused by being overweight relate to heart disease and diabetes. But cancer is also a risk, and not many people know this. A survey by the American Cancer Society recently showed that fewer than one in 20 people knew that being overweight increased their chance of getting cancer. Similarly, a European study asking men about the hazards of being too heavy showed that although four out of ten knew about heart disease or diabetes, cancer was not mentioned.

Just jumping on the scales or looking in the mirror does not necessarily tell you if you are overweight, or how overweight you are – though it might give you a strong clue or, forgive the pun, a heavy hint. The accurate measure is called the body mass index, or BMI. You can work out your BMI by measuring your weight, in kilograms, and your height, in metres; you then divide your weight by the square of your height. According to World Health Organization guidelines, if the answer comes out below 25 your weight is normal, if it is between 25 and 30 you are overweight, and if it is over 30 you are obese. Unfortunately the formula is a bit complicated, and most of us in the UK still think in imperial rather than metric measurements, so an example might help. If a man is 5 feet 7 inches tall and weighs 10½ stone, then his BMI is normal; if he weighs 12½ stone he will be overweight; and if he weighs 14½ stone then he will be obese.

The bad news is that the rate of obesity is rising rapidly in the UK and most of the Western world. Official government figures show that in 1980 only about seven in every 100 men and women were obese; by 2003 the number had more than tripled, to 22 out of every 100, and nearly 40 out of every 100 were overweight. So, overall, six out of ten people in the UK are either overweight or obese, and the numbers are still rising: obesity is an epidemic and a major health problem And the problem is not set to get any better, with the numbers of obese children also increasing alarmingly: another recent report has shown that in 1995 fewer than one in ten schoolchildren were obese, but by 2007 the number had almost doubled, to nearly one in five.

Cancer of the womb

The link between being overweight and developing cancer was first recognized in cancer of the womb (endometrial cancer). Each year more than 4,500 women in the UK will be told they have cancer of the womb, which makes it the fifth commonest cancer in women. Although most of those women will be cured, there are still about 900 deaths each year from the disease. So it is a major health problem, which at best needs major surgery, with a hysterectomy (and possibly radiotherapy), and at worst is fatal.

The evidence is that as many as four out of every ten cases of cancer of the womb are caused by being overweight. The cancer is usually diagnosed in older women, with an average age of 65, and studies have shown that a woman in her late fifties who is overweight or obese is five times more likely than other women to get endometrial cancer. But the risk begins to build up from an earlier age: if a woman is overweight at 21, she is three times more likely to develop womb cancer later in life; if a woman puts on weight between her twenties and fifties, increasing her body weight by one fifth or more during that time, then she doubles her risk of getting cancer of the womb. And the more weight gained, the greater the risk: if you are 22.5 kg or more overweight, then you are ten times more likely to get womb cancer than women of normal weight.

One other fact from the research is that putting on weight around your waist seems worse than putting it on at other parts of the body: that middle-aged spread could be bad news.

Scientists can also give us an explanation for why being too heavy increases a woman's risk of endometrial cancer. The female hormone, oestrogen, is mainly produced by the ovaries, but the body also makes oestrogen in fatty tissues, especially after the menopause when the ovaries have stopped working. The more fat you have, the more oestrogen you make. And oestrogen stimulates the cells in the lining of the womb to grow, and can overstimulate them to turn them into a cancer. Too much oestrogen for too long is dangerous, and the fatter you are the more oestrogen you will be making. This, I'm afraid, is the brutal truth.

Other cancers

And this same truth applies in breast cancer, where women who are past the menopause and overweight are once again at greater risk than those of the same age whose weight is in the normal range. Estimates suggest that almost one in ten breast cancers are caused by being overweight. Studies of large populations of women have shown that putting on 22.5 kg or more between being a teenager and reaching the menopause increases the risk of getting breast cancer by nearly 50 per cent, and even a much more modest increase of just a few pounds still makes breast cancer more likely. The good news is that these same studies have shown that women who are able to lose weight after the menopause actually reduce their chances of getting breast cancer. Age is the greatest single risk factor for breast cancer – the older you are, the more likely it is you will get it – but if you watch your weight and actually shed the pounds after the age of 50, then you are reducing the odds in your favour.

Men are also at risk from being too heavy. Studies suggest that about one in 20 prostate cancers are caused by being overweight; and of those cancers which affect both men and women, about one in ten colon cancers and as many as one in four cancers of the kidney are linked to being overweight or obese. There is also evidence that people who are obese and develop colon cancer, kidney cancer or cancer of the gullet (oesophagus) or pancreas are more likely to die from their cancer than people of normal weight.

In cancers other than breast and womb cancer, the explanation for why being overweight or obese puts you at increased risk is less certain. Hormone imbalance may be part of the problem: fatter people produce more insulin and insulin growth factor, as well as more sex steroids, which all have a role in controlling cell growth and development and so could lead to cancer formation. But although the underlying mechanism remains uncertain, the statistics are stark and inescapable: being overweight puts you at increased risk of getting a number of common cancers. Reduce your weight, and you reduce your risk.

The importance of exercise

How much we weigh is obviously linked to how much we eat, but it also depends on how much we exercise, how much physical activity we do to burn off the calories. Although few people realize it, regular exercise can help reduce our risk of getting cancer. More than 200 scientific studies have looked at the link between exercise and the chances of getting cancer, and the evidence of a benefit is overwhelming.

The largest body of evidence relates to colon cancer. Each year in the UK more than 20,000 men and women are diagnosed with this cancer of the large intestine, and despite recent improvements in treatment about half will eventually die of the disease. But studies have consistently shown that regular exercise reduces your chance of getting colon cancer by as much as 50 per cent. And regular exercise doesn't have to be a frantic workout at the gym every day or running the half-marathon before breakfast. Just a total of 30–40 minutes' brisk walking, five days a week, is enough to halve your likelihood of getting cancer of the colon.

Research has shown that taking a similar amount of exercise – 30 minutes' or more walking at a good pace, five times a week – will also reduce a woman's risk of getting breast cancer by between 20 and 40 per cent, and will reduce a smoker's risk of getting lung cancer by almost a third. For another group of cancers, including prostate cancer, skin cancer, testicular cancer and cancer of the womb, there is a strong suggestion that regular exercise means you're less likely to get any of these tumours, but it is difficult to put an accurate figure on the level of protection. It's also worth mentioning that none of the research that has been done on the link between exercise and cancer has been negative: in other words, there is no suggestion anywhere that more activity actually increases someone's risk of cancer.

Exactly why regular exercise can help prevent cancer remains uncertain. It could just be that people who are more physically active have a more healthy lifestyle generally, but there are also scientific findings showing that the levels of a number of growth factors circulating in the blood, which could cause cells to become cancerous, are reduced in people who are more active. In the case of colon cancer there is also the point that regular exercise helps move the contents of the bowel more quickly; this not only prevents constipation, but means that any traces of chemicals that could be cancer-forming (carcinogenic) are rapidly removed before they can do any harm.

Research on exercise and cancer has also shown that people who have had breast cancer or lung cancer can reduce the chance of the disease coming back by keeping active. Once again, the magic 30 minutes' or so walking, five days a week, is enough to make a difference, and to make a recurrence of the cancer less likely than in people who lead more sedentary lives.

There are two other encouraging points from the research. First, it is never too late to start exercising. Even if you are in your fifties or sixties and have been pretty inactive in the past, getting into the routine of some regular exercise can still make a difference. And second, there is no proof that very vigorous exercise has any extra benefit over just those few hours of brisk walking each week. So you don't have to push yourself to the limit.

Exercise helps us keep fit in other ways, and certainly reduces the risk of heart disease, which is an even bigger killer than cancer. It also improves the quality of life, reducing tiredness and boosting well-being and self-esteem. For some time now the government in the UK has recommended the brisk walking regime, 30 – 40 minutes, five days a week, or its equivalent, as a key part of a healthy lifestyle. But official figures suggest only a quarter of women and just over a third of men manage even this modest target. It doesn't take a lot to make a difference: walking up stairs rather than taking lifts or escalators, walking to the shops instead of getting into the car, or going for a turn round the park or along the canal towpath: a mile or two a day helps keep the cancer away!

HRT and 'the pill'

The link between cancer development and hormone replacement therapy (HRT) is a complex and controversial subject and is covered in Chapter 8 (p. 89).

There are two main types of contraceptive pill: combined preparations, which include both of the main female hormones, oestrogen and progestogen; and the progestogen-only tablet (sometimes called the mini-pill). A great many research studies have been done to look at the effects of taking these preparations on a woman's chances of getting cancer. The results are mixed, with a protective effect for some cancers and a slightly increased risk for others. Numerous reports have shown that taking the combined pill reduces a woman's likelihood of developing cancer of the womb (endometrial cancer) and cancer of the ovary. There is a suggestion from these reports that the longer a woman takes the pill the greater the protective effect, and that if a woman has taken it for about ten years then the protective benefit will last for another ten to 15 years after stopping it. Estimates on the degree of benefit vary, but a reduction in risk of about 50 per cent has been reported in a number of papers. There is also evidence that taking the pill may reduce the risk of developing bowel cancer, possibly by as much as 20 per cent. On the negative side, using the pill seems to be linked to an increased risk of cancer of the cervix (the neck of the womb) and breast cancer. There is no evidence linking the progestogen-only mini-pill to breast cancer development – indeed, some experts claim it may even slightly reduce the risk of the condition. For the combined pill there does seem to be a slight increase in breast cancer risk for younger women who take it for some time: the longer the time, the greater the risk.

So, for example, a woman of 25 who takes the combined pill for eight years will have about one and a half times the risk of getting breast cancer compared to a woman who has never taken the pill. But, as the chances of getting breast cancer at the age of 33 are very small, about one in 50,000, this means that the risk has still only increased to about one in 30,000: very small indeed. Once a woman stops taking the combined pill then her increased risk of breast cancer begins to reduce and has disappeared completely within ten years.

These reports have all focused on individual types of cancer, but the results published in a recent major study help to put the benefits and risks of taking the pill in context by looking at the effect on a very large population. This British study surveyed almost 750,000 women who had taken the pill and compared them with 340,000 women who had never taken it. Overall they found slightly fewer cancers among the women who had taken the pill, and concluded that it 'was not associated with an overall increase in cancer; indeed it may even produce a net public health gain'.

5

The world around us: cancer and the environment

Introduction

The world around us is constantly changing and cancer is getting more common. There is a temptation to link these two facts and look for changes in our environment as an explanation for cancers occurring. Sixty years ago we did not have nuclear power stations; since they first appeared the incidence of cancer in the UK has risen considerably, and many people are convinced that these two developments are cause and effect. On the other hand, 60 years ago virtually no one had a television; now almost all of us do, but the idea that radiation from our TV might cause cancer hasn't caught on.

Radiation is the main way the outside world affects our bodies. That radiation comes in two main types: ionizing and non-ionizing. Non-ionizing radiation includes ultraviolet rays, which we get in sunlight, radiofrequency fields, from mobile phones, and electromagnetic radiation, from things like overhead power lines. Ionizing radiation is 'radioactive' radiation, and we get this from a number of sources which may be either natural – coming from outer space and the ground beneath us – or artificial, from medical x-rays or nuclear power stations.

In this chapter we will look at some of these radiations in a bit more detail, but radiofrequency fields and electromagnetic radiation will be covered in Chapter 7, together with another environmental issue: air pollution.

Sunlight and cancer

When I first qualified as a doctor, almost 40 years ago, malignant melanoma was thought of as a rare cancer. Unfortunately times have changed, and it is now not only much more common but is also the fastest rising cancer in the UK. In 1995 there were fewer than 6,000 new cases in the UK; in 2004 there were almost 9,000, a rise of more than 40 per cent. It is also one type of cancer that often affects young people: one in five melanomas occur in people between the ages of 25 and 40. Although the cure rate is good for melanoma, the disease still causes nearly 2,000 deaths each year in the British Isles, and when a cure is possible it often involves a quite extensive operation, often with a skin graft, and some permanent scarring. So prevention is better than cure.

A major cause of malignant melanoma is over-exposure to sunlight, or more precisely to ultraviolet radiation. Ultraviolet (UV) radiation is that part of the sun's beams that makes us tan, giving us the bronzed healthy glow of film stars, TV celebrities and fashion models. It also causes our skin to age, losing its elasticity and becoming wrinkly. Over time it will also discolour our skin, giving it an unattractive yellowish tinge, often with brown patches and minute haemorrhages (which doctors call telangiectasia). It may make you look good, it may make you feel good, but a youthful tan comes with the risk that you will pay a heavy price for it in later life. The skin damage done by tanning doesn't go away: it just gradually builds up over the years as you get more ultraviolet radiation.

Ultraviolet radiation is at its most intense during the middle of the day on sunny days. And it's the sunshine that's the important thing, not the temperature; the warmth of the sun that we feel is due to harmless infra-red radiation, but if it's sunny, even on a cold day, then the damaging ultraviolet rays are still there. In fact they are even there when it's cloudy, although they are less intense.

This same UV radiation is what sunbeds and solaria use to produce a tan. Since sunbeds were first introduced in the late 1970s they have become extremely popular, with more and more young people using them to get a tan. This is despite the fact that, in a recent survey, more than half those going to solaria said they knew there was a cancer risk. And there is: it has been estimated that as many as one in four melanomas in young women and one in ten in young men are caused by sunbed use. A further worry is that these sunbeds are becoming more powerful and now produce rays more intense than the mid-day Mediterranean sun; although there is a British and European standard that puts a limit on this it is not legally enforceable, and as many as four out of every five commercial tanning machines are using more powerful UV radiation.

One recent news story graphically illustrates the dangers. A young woman of 29, living in the North West of England, died from widespread malignant melanoma. As a teenager she had used a sunbed twice a day for seven years. When she was 21 she learnt about the danger of skin cancer and stopped using the tanning beds. But seven years later she developed a melanoma and, despite treatment, could not be saved.

In general, skin damage and the risk of developing melanoma years later as a result of UV radiation is more likely for people with fair skin. The melanoma risk is increased if your skin burns in the sun, and the skin cancer risk is even higher if you get sunburnt in childhood.

Oh, and by the way, melanoma isn't the only skin cancer you can get from sunlight. UV radiation also causes basal cell carcinomas of the skin, known as rodent ulcers. These usually occur in later life and are often the result of long-term exposure to the elements – farmers, building workers and others who spend their lifetime out of doors are particularly at risk. There are no accurate figures for these particular cancers but estimates range from 50,000 – 150,000 new cases each year in the UK. The good news is that they are usually diagnosed when they are small, and are very easily treated by simple surgery or radiotherapy: they are usually completely curable. But, even so, they are a nuisance.

The UK Health Departments and Cancer Research UK offer excellent advice on how to reduce your chances of getting skin cancer in their Sun Smart campaign. The key messages are:

- Avoid going out in the sun between 11 a.m. and 3 p.m. or, if you do go out, keep in the shade.
- Make sure you never burn. Sunburn isn't just painful: it doubles your risk of skin cancer.
- If you are going out in strong sunlight, cover up with a t-shirt, hat and sunglasses. When the sun is at its peak, sunscreen isn't enough.
- Children should be especially careful. Young skin is delicate, and getting sunburn as a child is even more dangerous than getting it in later life.
- Use a sunscreen of factor 15 or above and apply it generously. And remember, reapply it often.

The Sun Smart campaign offers excellent advice, but sometimes the messages we get in the media can be confusing. Within weeks of reporting the death of the young woman who had habitually used sunbeds as a teenager, and using this to caution against the dangers of tanning shops and sunbathing, the papers were reporting that sunshine could reduce the risk of getting breast cancer. This was based on a study in the USA where almost 1,200 women, aged 55 or over, were given either supplements of vitamin D and calcium or an inactive placebo for four years. The researchers found that there were fewer cases of breast cancer among the women who took the supplements than among those who were on the placebo.

So what has that got to do with sunshine? Well, although we get some vitamin D in our food, in things like milk, eggs, green vegetables and oily fish, a lot of our supply of the vitamin is produced by our skin when it is exposed to sunlight. And that vitamin D is essential to keeping up our levels of calcium (which we need for healthy bones). So people who keep permanently out of the sun are likely to have lower levels of vitamin D, lower calcium levels and an increased risk of bone disease (especially a condition called rickets); in addition, as the new research suggests, they have an increased risk of breast cancer.

What are we to do? Do we risk getting melanoma, and other skin cancers, by going out in the sun, or stay in the shade and increase our chances of breast cancer? The answer, like nearly everything else in this book, is a matter of balance, of avoiding extremes. The Sun Smart campaign doesn't say 'never go out in the sun', but it does give good advice about avoiding too much sunlight or UV radiation. Similarly, the breast cancer researchers are not telling us to go and lie on Mediterranean beaches for 12 hours a day or use sunbeds seven days a week to avoid breast cancer; in terms of vitamin D production, a bit of sunshine goes quite a long way. So do let some sunshine into your life, but not too much.

Ionizing radiation

Living in a world where nuclear power stations and nuclear warheads exist, it is easy to believe that these significantly increase our exposure to ionizing radiation. But the estimates are that more than 80 per cent of the ionizing radiation we all get during our everyday lives comes from natural sources. Of the 16 per cent that comes from artificial, man-made sources, nearly all of this (15 of the 16 per cent) comes from medical tests and treatments, mainly from x-rays and CT scans. Only 1 per cent of our ionizing radiation exposure comes from the nuclear industry or nuclear weapons.

In terms of working out whether or not ionizing radiations cause cancer, a link can sometimes be made to specific events.

For example, after the Chernobyl nuclear disaster in 1986 there was an increase in the frequency of thyroid cancers in the surrounding area (but, surprisingly, no evidence of an increase in any other cancers). In general, however, the risks can only be calculated in relation to large populations rather than to individuals. So medical statisticians can estimate that certain levels of radiation might cause a certain number of additional cancers, but knowing whether any one individual's cancer was or was not due to that radiation is impossible to tell. For example, the calculation is that in the UK there may be as many as 700 cancers each year which have been caused by medical radiation from tests such as x-rays and CT scans, but there is no way of knowing, when someone does develop a cancer, whether this is due to having had x-rays or scans in the past. Incidentally, although the figure of 700 cancers each year may sound alarmingly high, it actually accounts for fewer than one in 1,200 cancers, and the official view is that the benefits that we all get from scans and x-rays far outweigh this statistically small risk.

Radon

From a cancer point of view, the most important source of ionizing radiation is a natural one: radon gas. Radon is a radioactive gas which is present in the ground and various rocks, and it seeps into our homes and makes up about half of all our exposure to ionizing radiation. Radon is particularly linked to the development of lung cancer, and the estimate is that about one or two in every 100 lung cancers could be due to radon exposure.

In England and Wales, radon levels are highest in Devon and Cornwall, a band across the south Midlands, central and western Wales and the Peak District. The official estimate is that as many as 100,000 homes may be built on land with an unsafe level of radon emissions. However, if your home is affected it doesn't mean you will have to move or have your house demolished; all that is needed are a few simple measures to improve the ventilation in the property and its foundations so that dangerous levels of radon cannot build up within the structure. In Northamptonshire there has been a very active programme to identify homes that might be at risk and to carry out modifications where necessary, and health officials think these measures might prevent as many as 14 lung cancers a year in the county.

Even if you live in an area with high radon levels, it may well be that your house is not actually affected. When you buy a property the environmental searches should tell you whether you are in a high radon area. The Health Protection Agency has a very helpful web site answering a range of questions on this subject; they also provide a free information pack, and can arrange measurements of the radon level in your home for a fee of about £40. Their contact details are in 'Useful addresses' at the end of this book.

6

Infection and cancer: cancer vaccines

Cervical cancer

At the beginning of this book I said that you cannot 'catch' cancer, so it might seem strange to have a chapter talking about infections as a cause of cancer. If you spend an evening in a crowded room with 20 other people, all of whom have heavy colds, then chances are that you will end up with a cold too. If you spend an evening in a crowded room with 20 people with cancer, there is no way you will get cancer from them. On the other hand, there are certain types of infection that can increase your chances of developing a cancer. Perhaps the easiest way to explain this is to look at an actual example.

The most common cancer where an infection has been shown to be a major cause of the disease is carcinoma of the cervix: cancer of the neck of the womb. Each year in the UK about 3,500 women will get cervical cancer. Worldwide the figure is a staggering half a million, with more than 250,000 women dying of the disease every year. We now know that more than four out of every five (80 per cent) cancers of the cervix are caused by an infection with a type of virus, a particular strain of the human papilloma virus, or HPV. This virus is carried from one person to another during sex. Most women who are sexually active are likely to develop an HPV infection at some time during their lives, however careful they are about their sexual hygiene and even if they only have one partner throughout their life. These infections usually have virtually no symptoms and so normally go completely unnoticed. There is no treatment for an HPV infection of the cervix and the condition will almost always go away by itself. But having an infection does increase your chance of getting cervical cancer, and the more episodes of infection the greater the risk. This means that women who are very sexually active, with multiple partners over time, and who have a higher chance of getting repeated HPV infections, have a greater risk of cervical cancer than other women.

What the HPV virus does is interact with a gene, or genes, in the cells on the surface of the cervix; this will cause mutations, and these can eventually lead to the development of a cancer. The first stage in this process is the appearance of pre-cancerous, benign changes in the appearance of the cells. These changes are called cervical intraepithelial neoplasia or, much more easily, CIN. Cells which have developed CIN can be seen under the microscope and detected as abnormal cells, although they are not yet cancerous. This is the basis of screening for cervical cancer, using the cervical smear test or its more recent update, liquid-based cytology. In both tests cells are scraped, or brushed, from the surface of the cervix and examined under the microscope. If CIN is detected then very simple treatment can be given that will prevent a cancer developing. Cervical screening allows the cancerous process to be nipped in the bud, and experts reckon that it saves more than 5,000 lives in the UK alone every year.

Having an HPV infection does not mean you will get a cancer of your cervix. Countless women will have an infection, or multiple infections, and never have any problem with cancer. But having an infection does put you at risk – if you don't get an HPV infection you almost certainly won't get cervical cancer; if you do, then you might. It's like saying that if you don't go on a train then you can't be in a train crash, but if you do, you may.

So by catching an HPV infection you are not catching a cancer, just increasing your risk. Your sexual partner is not actually giving you the cancer, but the infection you catch from him does mean that you have a chance of developing a cervical cancer, and you wouldn't have had that chance if you hadn't had the infection.

Vaccination

If we go back a couple of hundred years or so, cancer was much less common than it is today. The London Bill of Mortality for 1775 showed that just 54 people died from cancer in the capital that year. Today the figure would be more like 20,000. This difference is mainly because people are living far longer, and not dying from the other illnesses that were around at that time. Chief among these were the infectious diseases: going back to 1775, in that same year when just 54 Londoners died of cancer, 4,452 were victims of tuberculosis (TB), 2,700 died of smallpox and even measles claimed nearly 300 lives.

One of the great improvements in public health over the last 150 years has been the dramatic reduction in deaths from common infections like TB, smallpox and measles. The major reason for this improvement was the introduction of vaccination, which gave the body protection against these infectious diseases. Immunization programmes have proved a huge success in reducing the mortality from these infections, and in the case of smallpox and another scourge of the twentieth century, polio, have virtually wiped out the disease itself.

The idea that someone could one day invent a vaccine that would protect against cancer has always been one of medicine's Holy Grails. In reality, with so many different kinds of cancer, finding a single serum that could fight off the whole spectrum of malignant tumours was never going to be possible, even more so since cancer is not actually an infection and so vaccines wouldn't be effective.

Cervical cancer vaccines

Having said this, a major breakthrough in the last few years has been the development of two vaccines that can protect against the types of HPV infection that lead to cervical cancer. Clinical trials of these vaccines in young women between the ages of 15 and 26 show that they can prevent more than nine out of ten (over 90 per cent) of the herpes virus infections that lead to the changes of CIN, and so should protect against the development of cervical cancer. How long this protection lasts remains uncertain, simply because the vaccines haven't been around that long, but the benefit could last a lifetime.

This really is an amazing step forward. For the first time, there really is the likelihood of what is, in effect, a vaccination against cancer. By preventing the infection that causes it, the vaccines can prevent the cancer itself, offering the possibility of saving the lives of up to 1,400 women every year in the UK and 250,000 women around the world who die from cervical cancer every year.

The two vaccines are called Gardasil and Cervarix. At the time of writing, October 2007, the government has just announced that it is going to introduce a vaccination programme for girls from the age of 12 to 18. Vaccination involves a course of three injections, the second and third being given two and six months after the first. You have to have all three injections for the protection to be effective. The injections are given into the muscle in your upper arm or thigh. The only side effects are the possibility of soreness for a day or two at the site of the injection, with a bit of redness of the skin, and sometimes a brief rise in temperature, a short feeling of feverishness.

These vaccines are hugely important: for the first time women can actually be immunized against a common form of cancer. And there is a small bonus. The HPV virus is also the cause of most cancers of the vagina and the vulva, and of anal cancers

(cancers of the very last part of the bowel). So any woman who has one of the vaccines should be protected against these cancers as well.

Some questions

All this is extremely good news but, as ever, there are some questions and problems, and some practical issues.

Giving the vaccine only works as prevention, not a treatment; giving it after a woman has developed CIN, or a cervical cancer, is useless. The vaccines are a protection, not a cure. So when should they be given? The answer is, ideally before a woman begins to have sex. This would mean giving the vaccine to girls in their early teens, which is what is planned in the UK, but some experts have argued that it should be given at an even younger age, between eight and ten years old, since there is some evidence that the younger a girl is when she has the vaccine, the more effective it is.

Another question is whether young boys should also be vaccinated: this would reduce the risk of HPV infections being transmitted, and also give them protection from developing anal cancer – admittedly a rare type of cancer, but still a benefit.

There is also the concern that older women who have heard about the vaccine may stop going for their regular cervical screening checks, falsely believing that if they did develop a cancer of their cervix then the vaccine would be a cure. Continuing routine screening is essential for women who have not had the vaccine, and is still likely to be advisable for those who have, just as a 'belt and braces' protection against the much reduced risk of cervical cancer from HPV strains of virus not covered by the vaccines, or from other causes of cervical cancer. And should older women who have had a recent normal cervical smear test be offered the vaccine, to protect them in the future?

Then there is the hugely complicated moral and ethical dimension. Some people are worried that immunizing young girls against a common form of sexually transmitted infection would encourage them to be promiscuous (one Christian fundamentalist web site in the USA has dubbed the vaccine 'the sex jab'). For some cultures and some religious creeds, the idea of the vaccine could be difficult to come to terms with (there is another aspect to this, as the ethical opposition to the vaccine is most likely to come in those parts of the world where the risk of cervical cancer is greatest). Undoubtedly, debates will continue, probably often very vigorously and heatedly, for many years to come, before vaccination for cervical cancer finds its place in public health care worldwide.

Other cancers

As already mentioned, the same types of HPV virus which lead to cervical cancer also cause most cases of vaginal, vulval and anal cancer, so giving the anti-HPV vaccine Gardasil or Cervarix should help protect against these cancers. While this is good news, cancers of the vagina, vulva and anus are all quite rare, and altogether there are fewer than 2,000 new cases in the UK each year (just to put this figure in perspective, more than 900,000 people are diagnosed with cancer every year in the UK).

Another vaccine that has been available for more than 20 years is the hepatitis B vaccine. This protects against a particular type of viral infection of the liver that may lead to primary liver cancer: hepatocellular carcinoma. This cancer is very uncommon in the UK, but worldwide it is the third biggest cause of cancer deaths, with more than half a million people dying every year. In the UK the small number of cases does not justify a mass vaccination programme, but in countries where the disease is widespread, like Taiwan, hepatitis B vaccination has led to a major fall in the number of people getting this type of cancer. Incidentally, it is important to remember that hepatitis B is only linked to primary liver cancer, and not to secondary cancers which have spread to the liver from growths in other parts of the body (like the breast, the bowel or the lung). Unfortunately there is no vaccine to protect against these liver secondaries, which are far more common than the primary hepatocellular carcinomas.

Viral infections are known to be a factor in the development of some other cancers. People with HIV–AIDS have a greater than normal risk of developing a number of cancers, including cervical cancer, a cancer of the lymph glands called non-Hodgkin's lymphoma, and a cancer which most often appears on the skin, called Kaposi's sarcoma. Burkitt's lymphoma, another cancer of the lymph glands, and a cancer affecting the lining of the back of the nose, nasopharyngeal cancer, are also related to viral infections. Treating these infections reduces the cancer risk, but at the moment there is no prospect of vaccines to protect against getting the infection in the first place.

When it comes to the really common cancers – breast cancer, lung cancer, prostate cancer and bowel cancer – there is no evidence of infections increasing the chance of getting any of these growths, so vaccination has no future in their prevention. For these cancers we have to look for other means of prevention.

Vaccination: what can you do?

The Department of Health for England and Wales is bringing in a programme of HPV vaccination for girls aged 12 to 13, starting in September 2008. It has also announced that there will be a two-year 'catch-up' campaign for girls aged up to 18 years, starting in autumn 2009. The Scottish Executive has said it hopes to introduce such a programme in late 2008. In the meantime, HPV vaccine is available privately, at a cost of between

£400 and £600. Whether there will be the offer of 'catch-up' vaccination for older teenage girls remains uncertain. Hepatitis B vaccination is available for people who have been in contact with the disease or are at risk of being exposed to it. With all this in mind you should:

- continue your normal cervical screening if you are a woman between the ages of 25 and 64;
- think about whether you would like to have the HPV vaccine if it becomes available on the NHS (or even sooner, if you can afford to pay for it) if you are a woman who has had a recent normal cervical screening test;
- be thinking about whether your children should have the vaccine, if you have young daughters;
- make sure you have hepatitis B vaccination if you have been in contact with the disease or are at risk of coming into contact with it.

7

Some myths about what causes cancer

Introduction

Why me? Why did I get cancer? This is one of the most common questions that people ask when they find they have a cancer. It is very natural to want an explanation, to understand why it is that you have got the disease. But in many instances it is still a question that doctors cannot answer. For most cancers there is no definite cause and effect, nothing that we can be sure directly led to the cancer appearing. But for many people that information vacuum is difficult to come to terms with – they really need a reason why their cancer came. Over the years countless explanations have been put forward to meet this need, theories that range from the completely hair-brained to the really quite reasonable. Some of these gain more acceptance than others, even though there is no scientific evidence to support them, and become widely believed cancer myths.

To try and catalogue all these different beliefs, which are often held with a passionate conviction by many people, would take a book of its own. So in this chapter I have just selected a personal top ten examples to look at in a bit more detail.

Mobile phones and phone masts

One of the things that modern-day society is very worried about as a possible cause of cancer is the ever-increasing use of mobile phones. The scientific community is well aware of this concern and numerous studies have been done, and are still continuing, to try to find out whether there is a risk. One problem here is the timescale. I can remember the first mobile phone I ever used: it was in about 1992 and belonged to the hospital, and whichever doctor was on call took it home at weekends. The phone was about the size of a brick and weighed only slightly less – when I went shopping it needed its own carrier bag. The point of this story is that mobile phones have only been in common use for just over ten years, and given the time it takes some cancers to develop, it will probably be another ten years before we can be absolutely sure that they carry little or no cancer risk. So far, despite many people's fears and occasional media scares, there is no evidence that there is a danger.

The one possible link – and even here the evidence is very weak – is to a very slightly increased risk of getting something called an acoustic neuroma. This is an uncommon tumour affecting the main nerve of the ear. In fact, acoustic neuromas are not cancers, they are benign tumours – so newspaper headlines proclaiming that researchers may have found a link between mobile phone use and brain cancer are wrong on two counts: acoustic neuromas occur near to, but not in, the brain, and they are not cancers. But to explain that this still slight possibility of an increased risk relates to a benign tumour of the acoustic nerve is probably too much for most journalists to cope with, and anyway it doesn't make nearly such a good story.

So, mobile phones and cancer, the verdict? We will have to wait another decade or more to be sure, but so far the evidence is: no evidence.

Closely linked to the phones themselves are the masts that are used to relay their signals. Cancer is very common, and if there are people living near to a mobile phone mast then inevitably, at some time, one or more of them will get cancer – that is a statistical fact, and not the result of the presence of the phone mast. Similarly, once in a while there will be a cluster of people with cancer near to a particular mast, just as clusters of cancers occur in the rest of the population. Once again, this is just a normal statistical probability. Studies have looked at this very carefully, and the evidence is that there is no increased cancer risk from having a phone mast close to your home or your school. But a lot of people remain convinced that there is a danger, even accusing the government of a conspiracy with the phone industry to hide the real facts.

Overhead power cables

Many people are worried that living close to overhead electricity power lines might increase their chances of getting cancer. These cables produce electromagnetic fields which do send small electric currents through our bodies when we are near them. But those currents are actually smaller than the normal electrical impulses that run through our nerves to control things like our breathing and heartbeat. So the level of 'artificial' electrical activity from power lines is lower than the natural level in our bodies. Also, there is no clear explanation for why these electromagnetic fields might lead to cancer developing; there is no biological process to link the two.

Despite the unlikelihood that there could be a risk, a lot of research has been done on this subject and all the evidence is that there is no risk for adults. But one very detailed British study, which reported in 2005, found that children living within 200 metres of these cables were almost twice as likely to develop leukaemia as children living further away. At first sight this sounds quite dramatic, but the actual number of cases of leukaemia in the study was very small: childhood leukaemia is quite an uncommon disease and relatively few people live close to power lines, and so it was difficult to be sure whether or not the result was just down to chance rather than a real relationship between the cables and the leukaemia. Even if there were a true cause-and-effect link, this would only account for about one in every 100 cases of childhood leukaemia, which is the same as saying that five children a year in the UK might develop leukaemia because they live near to power cables. But the evidence is far from certain, and for adults living close to power cables, or anyone living more than 400 metres from the cables, there is absolutely no suggestion of any cancer risk.

Dairy foods and breast cancer

My homework last weekend was to check exam questions for our fourth-year medical students' end of year exam in oncology. One of the questions was 'Which of the following does NOT increase a woman's risk of breast cancer?' The correct answer in the list of five options was 'Regularly eating dairy products'. The fact that this was included in an undergraduate examination is a sign of just how powerful and prevalent this particular myth is. Many women believe with a passionate conviction that eating butter, cheese and yoghurt or drinking milk causes breast cancer, and have radically altered their diets to cut out all traces these items. But it is a myth.

So why is this belief so widespread? Milk is rich in fat, and with modern-day farming methods it often contains traces of various hormones, and toxins from pesticides and other chemicals. In theory, any of these might lead to a risk of breast cancer. This possibility is increased by the circumstantial evidence that in countries where people eat fewer dairy products breast cancer is less common. These factors, combined with the anecdotal accounts of some women who have had remissions of their cancer after a change in their diet, cutting out dairy products, have led to a number of books, articles and web sites passionately arguing that milk, butter and cheese are high risk factors for breast cancer and should be avoided at all costs.

Those arguments can sound very convincing. But countless scientific studies, using a variety of different epidemiological methods, have failed to prove the link. In the last three years there have been at least three major reviews of the scientific evidence on this subject published in leading medical journals; all agreed that although more than 50 studies had been carried out, there was no epidemiological evidence to support a link between the consumption of dairy products and an increased risk of breast cancer. There are people who will see this as a scientific conspiracy to hide the real truth from us, and who will continue to believe either that dairy products cause breast cancer, or that giving up dairy products can make a cancer go away, or both. But from a medical and scientific point of view those beliefs have no real evidence to support them.

Injuries

Sticks and stones may break my bones – but they won't give me cancer. Many people believe that their cancers were caused by earlier injuries: bumps or bruises, falls or fractures. This belief is particularly common among women with breast cancer and young people who develop bone tumours. Typical stories are 'I was looking after my two-year-old grandson and when I picked him up he kicked my breast. A month later I found a lump there which turned out to be cancer' or 'I was kicked on the shin playing football and got a nasty bruise. Six weeks later they discovered I had a cancer there.' It seems quite logical that if you have an injury to part of your body, and a short time later a cancer is discovered at that site, then the two must be related: cause and effect. But there is no evidence whatsoever that this is the case.

One factor that is important here is the timescale. As we have seen (p. 16), nearly all cancers take a long time to develop, usually a period of years between the first cancerous change and the time there is a lump big enough to be diagnosed. So an injury a few days, weeks or even months before a cancer is discovered simply could not have caused it to happen: the cancer would have been growing there long before the trauma occurred. Almost always, what has happened is that because of the injury the person has become more aware of that part of the body, has watched and examined it more closely, and discovered a lump or noticed a pain or swelling that hadn't been recognized before. This alerted him or her to the fact that there was something wrong and led to the cancer being diagnosed. In other words, the injury was a coincidence: it just happened to damage that part of the body where the cancer already was, but did not cause it in the first place.

Stress

A few years ago one of my colleagues found herself at a dinner, sitting next to the chief executive of a multi-national corporation. By way of conversation she asked him, 'What do you do about stress among your senior executives?'

'I make sure they get as much as possible!' was the answer.

Whether his unsympathetic response would be likely to increase or decrease his employees' chances of getting cancer is controversial. As long ago as 1893, in one of the first scientific reports looking at possible causes of cancer, H. L. Snow recorded that many of the patients had 'a general liability to the buffets of ill-fortune'. Bringing things up to date, in 2001 a UK survey showed that four out of ten women thought stress was a major cause of breast cancer. This view that there is a link between stressful life events and cancer is a popular one, and people will often link the onset of their cancer to the death of a partner, the loss of a job, a divorce or some other major emotional upset. In scientific terms it has been shown that stress reduces the efficiency of our immune systems, and there is also the likelihood that people under stress might take to smoking, drinking or over-eating to help cope, all of which might increase their cancer risk.

Once again, researchers have done numerous studies trying to measure stress and see whether it might lead to cancer. The evidence is conflicting: there are a handful of studies that suggest there could be a link, but most can find no difference in the history of stress among people with cancer and the rest of the population. There have even been a couple of studies in breast cancer suggesting that higher stress levels might actually reduce a woman's chances of getting the disease. Stress is an emotive subject, and there is no doubt that being overstressed is not good for our general health, but as far as cancer is concerned there is still no proof of a link between emotional distress and our risk of developing the disease.

Abortion and breast cancer

During pregnancy there are huge changes in a woman's hormone levels, and these will have a marked effect on her breasts. It has been suggested that if this natural cycle of shifting hormonal patterns is interrupted by an abortion, whether that occurs naturally (as a miscarriage) or artificially (as an induced termination), this could be damaging and might even trigger the development of a breast cancer.

This possibility has been extensively researched since the 1950s. The early studies gave conflicting results, some suggesting that women who had experienced an abortion were more likely to get breast cancer, and others showing no increase in their risk. Many of these reports were based on unreliable methods, either surveying too few women or using sampling and questioning methods that introduced unintentional biases into the results. More recent, larger, better studies have given a much more consistent answer, showing no link between abortion and breast cancer. The largest of these surveys, involving more than a million Danish women, was published during the 1990s, and using results from this and many other trials, in 2003 an international panel of experts reviewing all the evidence concluded that having had an abortion did not increase a woman's chances of getting breast cancer. This message was reinforced in 2007 when a large study in the USA published its findings, once again showing no increase in risk.

Abortion is a highly emotionally charged subject and has very intense religious and political overtones. There are still people and organizations that remain convinced that having a miscarriage, or more especially an induced termination, leads to breast cancer. The internet bristles with web sites proclaiming this as a fact, and every so often newspaper or magazine articles will try and resurrect the argument. But putting passion, religious conviction and political persuasion to one side, the overwhelming scientific evidence is, once again, that having an abortion does not mean a woman is more likely to get breast cancer.

Vasectomy and prostate cancer

There have been a number of research studies that have suggested that having a vasectomy may increase a man's risk of developing prostate cancer, but there have also been other studies where no such increase in risk was found. In the early 1990s the World Health Organization held a meeting of experts to examine all the data, and they concluded that there was no evidence of a link between vasectomy and prostate cancer.

This seems a very reasonable conclusion and is supported by two other factors: first, there is no biological explanation for why having a vasectomy might have an effect on the prostate gland – there is no explanation for a link between 'the cut' and the cancer – and, second, even in those studies that suggested an increased risk, the level of risk was very small, with the chances of a man getting prostate cancer being increased by only 1 or 2 per cent (another way of putting this is that if you had a group of 10,000 men, half of whom had had a previous vasectomy and half of whom hadn't, then in the vasectomized men 102 would be likely to get prostate cancer, compared to 100 in the non-vasectomized group). It has been suggested that these very tiny differences could be due to factors other than the vasectomy itself: for example, one theory is that men who have a vasectomy tend to be more health conscious and so might also be more likely to go for prostate cancer screening, which might detect the disease more often. So overall the evidence is that there is no link.

Air pollution

A recent survey showed that four out of ten people thought that air pollution was more likely to cause lung cancer than smoking a pack of 20 cigarettes a day, underlining a widely held belief that the two are linked.

To some extent this goes along with the idea that we live in a more polluted world nowadays. I'm old enough to remember the choking filth of London smogs of 50 years ago. (Incidentally, fans of conspiracy theories will be delighted to know that in the 1950s the government suppressed a report by the UK Medical Research Council on the health hazards of smog, including lung cancer, because it would cause too much public alarm.) Happily, air pollution has reduced very considerably in the UK and most other Western countries over the last few decades. But very large studies in Europe and the USA have shown that, despite this improvement, long-term exposure to high levels of pollution – for example, living next to a busy main road in a heavily industrialized area for about ten to 15 years – can increase someone's risk of lung cancer: the greater the level of pollution and the longer the exposure to it, the greater the risk. But even with quite high levels of pollution from traffic fumes and factory smokestacks, someone's risk of lung cancer would only increase by about 10 per cent; to put it another way, overall about 30 out of every 1,000 people in the UK get lung cancer, and in heavily polluted areas that figure might rise to 33 out of every 1,000. In the UK, air pollution from vehicle exhausts and heavy industry probably causes about three out of every 100 cases of lung cancer. This may sound alarming, but it is still a very small number compared to the 95 or so cases out of every 100 that are due to smoking.

Underarm deodorants and breast cancer

The idea that using underarm deodorants or antiperspirants might increase a woman's risk of breast cancer began as an internet rumour but was then picked up by scientists who decided to look into the truth of the matter. The theory behind the story was that the deodorants might contain chemicals which could lead to breast cancer, and that these chemicals could either be absorbed through the skin or get into the blood stream through small cuts or scratches if a woman regularly shaved her underarms.

One scientist in particular seems to have made it her life's work to try and prove the point, and has published a number of reports in recent years showing that ingredients such as parabens or calcium in deodorants and antiperspirants can be detected in breast tissue following their use. Other scientists and medical experts have been highly critical of her research methods, citing such things as the small numbers of samples in her studies and the fact that she does not use a control group to compare her results with samples from women who don't use these products (other studies have suggested the same 'dangerous' chemicals are present in the breast tissue of women who don't use deodorants). However, this is a good story, and every time she publishes a new report at least one of the UK's national daily papers will feature her work and re-run the scare story of the link between using underarm deodorants and the risk of breast cancer. But all the major cancer research organizations have looked at this question and the so-called research on the subject, and they all agree that there is no good evidence for an increased cancer risk.

Hair dyes and tints

Surveys have suggested that in the UK as many as one in three women regularly use hair dyes and tints, and, perhaps rather surprisingly, as many as one in ten men over the age of 40 also use them. Over the years there have been stories linking hair dyes and colourants to bladder cancer, breast cancer, leukaemia and cancers of the lymphatic system (lymphomas). These originally stem from laboratory experiments done more than 30 years ago, which showed that some chemicals, in some dyes, could cause damage to cells grown in cultures and could also cause cancers in mice. As a result these chemicals were banned from use in cosmetic materials.

Since then many studies have been done to see whether people who regularly use hair dyes are at greater risk of getting cancer. In 2005 the *Journal of the American Medical Association* published an analysis of all the available information, and this concluded that there was no good evidence of an increased cancer risk. Some scientists still have slight concerns about some of the chemicals used in permanent hair dyes; however, the evidence linking their use to the development of cancers is very weak, so if you want to be as safe as possible then using a semi-permanent product is the answer.

8

Chemoprevention: drugs to stop cancer forming

Chemoprevention

Wouldn't it be great if you could just take a pill that would stop you getting cancer? There are plenty of internet sites and quack doctors that would like to persuade you this is possible, at a price, but in the real world of scientific, evidence-based medicine it largely remains a dream for the future. But in a few cancers some progress in chemoprevention – the use of drugs to stop cancers developing – is being made, and this chapter explores what has been achieved so far.

When I was a young medical student, way back in the 1960s, I remember being quite amazed when I came across a chapter in one of my textbooks on 'Drugs to treat cancer'. I had no idea that there were such drugs: if they existed, why wasn't cancer cured? Today we have many more anti-cancer drugs than we did 40 years ago, and many more cancers are cured as a result. But unfortunately cures are still not universal and the drugs, and other treatments, don't always work. One of the many reasons for this is that most of the drugs used to treat cancer have quite powerful side effects, and sometimes these limit their useful-ness, restricting the doses that can be given or the length of time for which they can be taken, so that not everyone will get a benefit from them.

This problem with side effects is a major issue in using drugs to prevent cancer. The whole idea of prevention means fit, healthy people taking tablets or medicines over a long period, often many years, in order for them to work. If those compounds are going to cause serious side effects then that is simply not acceptable. This is the big difficulty: most of the drugs used to treat cancer are too toxic to use in cancer prevention. If someone has a life-threatening cancer then it is entirely right and proper to prescribe powerful drugs to treat the condition – even if they might have unpleasant, or even dangerous, side effects – if they offer the chance of a cure or a considerable increase in life-expectancy. But to use those same drugs on a normal population of well people, most of whom never will get cancer, and expose them to the risk of serious complications, is utterly unacceptable. So any drug used for cancer prevention has to be extremely safe, and that is a major hurdle to overcome.

Despite this handicap of having to ensure drug safety, some progress has been made in chemoprevention in three of the major cancers: breast cancer, bowel cancer and prostate cancer.

Breast cancer

Tamoxifen is a hormonal drug that first appeared in the 1970s. Although it was initially intended as a treatment for infertility, it rapidly became clear that it was a major breakthrough in the treatment of breast cancer. As well as being an active drug against the cancer, it offered the bonus of appearing to have no serious side effects (although a minority of women taking the drug did have troublesome menopausal symptoms, such as hot flushes, night sweats and loss of concentration). Because of this success specialists began to wonder whether tamoxifen could actually be given to prevent breast cancer. In due course clinical trials were set up where women who were thought to have a high risk of getting breast cancer, because of their family history of the disease, were offered either tamoxifen or an inactive placebo.

The results of the trials have been mixed. Some have shown a benefit, with fewer breast cancers occurring in the women taking tamoxifen, while others have shown no difference. Statisticians have tried putting all the different results together and looking at them in what is called a meta-analysis. This suggests that overall tamoxifen might reduce the chances of a breast cancer developing by up to 40 per cent (in other words, for every 100 breast cancers that would have occurred before, only 60 will occur if the women at risk take tamoxifen).

While this sounds like good news, the picture is further complicated by the fact that, over the time the trials have been in progress, it has become clear that tamoxifen is not quite as safe as people thought at first, and with its longer-term use two important, potentially serious, problems have emerged: it may increase a person's chances of developing thromboses and blood clots, and it can very occasionally lead to the development of cancer of the womb. For women who need tamoxifen as an essential part of the treatment for their breast cancer, these risks (which affect only a small minority of patients) are far outweighed by the benefits, but for otherwise fit and healthy women who are taking tamoxifen long term to try and prevent a breast cancer appearing, the balance shifts and the safety concern over the side effects is far greater.

At the present time doctors have responded differently to these findings: in the USA they have produced firm guidelines for when tamoxifen should be used for certain groups of women who are at very high risk of developing breast cancer, whereas in the UK no such guidance has been issued, with specialists being less convinced about the value of the drug, and also concerned about its safety in this particular population of well women.

Research in the field of hormone treatment to prevent breast cancer is still ongoing. One study is looking at a drug called raloxifene, which is similar to tamoxifen and has been used to prevent osteoporosis (thinning of the bones in older women). There is some evidence that raloxifene might be effective and it has the benefit of a better safety profile than tamoxifen, with no risk of thrombosis or womb cancer. Another group of drugs are called aramotase inhibitors. These are effective treatments for breast cancer, and once again have fewer side effects than tamoxifen; their major limitation is that they only work in women who are past the menopause, so they are not suitable for breast cancer prevention in younger women.

Another limitation that affects all types of hormonal measures to prevent breast cancer is that they will only stop those cancers which are hormone-dependent (so-called oestrogen-positive or ER+ cancers) from developing. These are breast cancers that rely on a supply of the female hormone, oestrogen, in the blood stream to encourage their growth. Overall, these make up about two-thirds of all breast cancers, but this still means there is a substantial minority of breast cancers that won't be inhibited by drugs like tamoxifen or raloxifene and would still appear even if these drugs were given.

Drug prevention of breast cancer provides an opportunity to mention a couple of the problems linked to getting hard evidence for what is best. At the time of writing, doctors in the USA have for some time been planning a major clinical trial that should answer a lot of the remaining questions surrounding this issue: the STELLAR trial. This will involve some 13,000 women, and with such a large group should give some very reliable results. But it will take at least ten years to complete and will cost a quite staggering $100 million to run. So not only will we have to wait more than a decade for any answers, but the sheer expense of doing the research is raising questions over whether the study will be possible. At the moment the future of the STELLAR trial hangs in the balance. Getting answers in cancer prevention, answers that can be believed, is neither quick nor cheap.

The other side of this coin is the anxiety that some hormone preparations could actually increase a woman's risk of breast cancer. The key culprit here is hormone replacement therapy (HRT). A huge amount of research has been done to try to work out whether or not taking HRT is a cancer risk, and the answers aren't simple. The first thing to say is that for women under the age of 50 there is no evidence of an increased risk of getting breast cancer if they take HRT, so for younger women there isn't a problem. When it comes to looking at the possible dangers for women of 50 or over, you need to bear in mind that there are two different types of HRT: one relies on small doses of the female hormone, oestrogen, on its own (oestrogen-only HRT), while the other adds in a second hormone, progesterone, and this is called combined HRT.

The results of clinical trials involving literally millions of women show that taking either oestrogen-only or combined HRT in the short term, for a year or less, doesn't seem to affect the chances of getting breast cancer. With longer periods of medication there is a risk, and this increases with time. Let's use real figures to put this in perspective. For every 1,000 women between the ages of 50 and 64 who have never taken HRT, 32 would be expected to develop breast cancer. If they had all taken oestrogen-only HRT for five years this figure would rise to 34, and if they had taken it for ten years the number would be 37. For combined HRT the figures would be an extra six cases after five years' HRT, and 19 more after ten years. At first sight this suggests that oestrogen-only HRT is a lot safer; the problem is that taking the oestrogen-only preparation increases the risk of developing womb cancer by about 50 per cent and may also increase, slightly, a woman's chances of getting cancer of the ovary. Because of these hazards oestrogen-only HRT is usually only given to women who have had a hysterectomy. Just to confuse things further, there is some good news about HRT and cancer, and that is that some trials have suggested it reduces the risk of getting bowel cancer, although the evidence for this is less well defined than the breast cancer side of the story.

So for women over 50, taking HRT does increase your breast cancer risk, and the longer you taker it the greater that risk becomes, so that after ten years on combined HRT your risk has gone up by more than 50 per cent. On the other hand this still means that your chance of getting the disease before 65 are only about one in 20, compared with about one in 30 if you hadn't taken HRT; taking the hormones has reduced the odds that you could have a breast cancer, but it certainly doesn't mean that you definitely will.

And most women don't take HRT for fun. Usually it is given to help cope with menopausal symptoms, like hot flushes, night sweats, loss of libido, vaginal dryness, and so on. For some women these are very minor problems, but for others they can be hugely distressing, even driving them to the brink of suicide. So, at the end of the day, whether or not to have HRT is a matter of weighing up the risks and the benefits – if the hot flushes are ruining your life, making you clinically depressed and raising thoughts of ending it all, then a slight increase in the possibility of getting breast cancer is a minor consideration and HRT is the answer, but if your symptoms aren't really much bother then avoid it. If you are concerned and in doubt, the thing to do is to have a chat with your family doctor, who can help you weigh up your individual pros and cons so that you can reach an agreed, and informed, decision on what to do.

Bowel cancer

Aspirin has been around as an all-purpose painkiller for the last hundred years, but for some time now researchers have wondered whether it could also stop cancer. The thinking behind this is that many cancers produce abnormal amounts of two chemicals, cyclooxygenase-2 (COX-2) and prostaglandin, which appear to be essential for them to grow. Aspirin interferes with the production of these compounds and reduces their level in the tissues. So giving aspirin might stop the process of cancer development and growth. Support for this idea comes from a number of studies that were actually looking for another possible benefit of aspirin: its ability to reduce heart disease and strokes. These trials looked at a large number of volunteers who were given daily doses of aspirin for a number of years, and then did long-term checks on their health to see if they had fewer strokes and heart attacks than a similar group of people who had not taken aspirin. Although mainly designed to look at the frequency of heart disease and strokes, these studies also looked at other medical problems, including cancer. One of the largest of the trials involved more than 5,000 British doctors, two-thirds of whom took aspirin for between five and six years while one third did not, beginning in 1978–9. They were then followed up for the next 20 years and all their health problems recorded.

The results of these and other epidemiological studies have suggested that aspirin might reduce the risk of a number of cancers, but the strongest evidence of a benefit has been for bowel cancer. Overall the results do show that taking aspirin reduces the likelihood of getting a cancer of the large bowel, the colon or rectum. But this doesn't mean that rushing out now and swallowing two aspirin tablets will stop you getting one of these tumours. The evidence is that aspirin has to be taken every day for somewhere between five and ten years to have any effect, and it is only some years after this that a reduction in the number of cancers shows up (which reflects the fact that most bowel cancers take a decade or more to develop). Even so, since some of the research that has been done suggests that the risk of getting a bowel cancer could be halved by taking daily aspirin, you may think that doctors and health authorities ought to be advertising the fact and suggesting we should all be doing this. But there are problems.

First of all, no one is sure what dose of aspirin is needed to have a protective effect. The evidence suggests that low doses don't work and that quite a high dose is necessary – but what the right dose is remains unknown. Nor is anyone sure how long you need to take it: certainly for a number of years, but how many years? Nobody knows. And then we come back to side effects: taking an occasional aspirin for a headache or muscular aches and pains is fine, but taking regular daily tablets at quite high doses greatly increases the risk of complications like stomach and duodenal ulcers and the risk of bleeding from the lining of the stomach and the gut, bleeding which can sometimes be sudden, serious and even fatal.

So although overall the evidence is that regular aspirin reduces the risk of getting bowel cancer, the fact is that the degree of risk reduction, the degree of protection, varies considerably between different studies and there is total uncertainty over how much of the drug you should take, and for how long. The risk of serious side effects means that the jury is still out as to whether this could be a useful approach to cancer prevention.

Aspirin belongs to a family of drugs called non-steroidal anti-inflammatory agents (NSAIDs for short). These are widely used to treat conditions like arthritis and rheumatism. A number of NSAIDs have been tested to see whether they could prevent cancer. Again, some studies do show a benefit, but the same problems over dose, length of treatment and risk of side effects that have limited progress with aspirin apply to these other NSAIDs as well.

Although the possible protective effect of NSAIDs has been studied most extensively in bowel cancer prevention, other cancers have also been looked at. A number of reports have suggested that regular aspirin or other NSAIDs can reduce the risk of breast cancer, lung cancer, prostate cancer, cancer of the gullet (the oesophagus), cancer of the stomach and cancer of the ovary. But again, the evidence isn't absolutely conclusive, and the same questions over dose, the length of time the drugs need to be taken and that worry about side effects mean that the experts still aren't recommending the widespread use of NSAIDs as a way of preventing cancer. Balancing out medical risks and benefits is always extremely difficult, but doctors will always put people's safety first and, until these questions have been fully answered and the true benefits and risks are known, then the advice is likely to be cautious. So we're some way away from having aspirin in the tap water to stop us getting cancer!

Prostate cancer

This brings us back to hormones again. Just as about two-thirds of all breast cancers need a supply of oestrogen to support their growth, more than nine out of ten prostate cancers rely on the male hormone, testosterone, in order to develop and flourish. If the supply of that hormone to the cancer is reduced in any way then the tumour will stop growing and the cancer cells will begin to die off.

The chance of a man developing prostate cancer is about one in six, so it is a common problem – in fact, it is now the most common cancer in men in the UK, having overtaken lung cancer a year or two ago. But it usually only affects older men: it is rare below the age of 60, and it most often affects those in their seventies and eighties. As a rule it is also the case that the older a man is when he gets prostate cancer, the more slow-growing the condition will be, so that many men who are first diagnosed in their late seventies or eighties will have very few problems and need very little treatment, being able to live in peace with their cancer.

Also, in contrast to breast cancer, it is quite difficult to identify a specific population that might be at a high risk of developing prostate cancer. So any attempt at prevention has to be widely based rather than targeting a selected group of individuals.

Despite these various limitations, a lot of work has been done looking at a hormonal drug called finasteride, which reduces the level of testosterone in the blood. The largest study to date looked at over 18,000 men in the USA who were aged over 55; half were given finasteride and half a placebo. The results showed that men taking finasteride got fewer prostate cancers: about one in four men taking the placebo developed the disease, whereas in those on the hormone the figure was one in five.

A reduction of one fifth may not sound too dramatic, but in the UK this would translate into over 6,000 fewer cases of prostate cancer each year. But the trial was not all good news. Although there were fewer prostate cancers in the men taking finasteride, there was a suggestion that the tumours that did occur in this group were more aggressive and more dangerous. There was also, again, the problem of side effects, particularly relating to a loss of sexual potency and impotence in the men taking the hormone.

Trials are ongoing with other drugs related to finasteride but at the moment the available evidence means that, once more, the jury is still out as far as drug prevention of prostate cancer is concerned. There are certainly no plans to introduce the offer of mass finasteride-dosing in the over 55s as a protective measure. But it is just possible that it could be considered on an individual basis if a man in late middle age was known to have a set of risk factors that put him at extremely high risk of developing the disease.

So what do you do?

So for the population as a whole, taking a pill to stop getting cancer remains a fantasy. But for a carefully selected group of people, who for one reason or another are clearly at far greater risk of developing breast cancer or prostate cancer, then hormonal treatment to try and reduce their risk might be an option, and it might just be considered for some people with a high risk of getting bowel cancer. But the weighing up of those risks, the balancing of the possible benefits and hazards of taking a prolonged course of preventive drug treatment, should only be done with the help and advice of expert medical opinion. This is a very complicated area, not without its risks, and is not something that people should contemplate without detailed guidance and counselling from their doctors.

9

Screening for cancer

Screening for cancer saves more than 7,000 lives every year in the UK. So what is it? Screening involves looking at a group of people who appear to be perfectly healthy to see whether they have a cancer, or a condition that might turn into a cancer. The aim is to pick up the problem at its earliest stage, when a cancer can still be prevented, or if a cancer has developed to treat it before it can spread and do serious harm.

There is no reliable way of screening just for 'cancer' as a whole. Despite claims on the internet, there is no sure method of testing to see whether someone has, or has not, got a cancer somewhere in his or her body. Even if we did have such a test it would only be of limited value. Certainly it would be good news if you had the test and it was negative, giving you the all clear. But if it came back positive, lots more tests would be needed to find out just where the cancer was, which organ was actually affected. What we do have are a number of tests that can be used to look for specific types of cancer, in certain parts of the body. These are cancer of the cervix (the neck of the womb), the breast and the large bowel (the colon and rectum). There is also the controversial question of screening for prostate cancer.

Cancer screening involves looking at people of certain ages in the population as a whole. To make it worthwhile, a number of criteria have to be met. Among the more important of these are that the condition you are looking for is a common health problem, that there is a reliable test to detect it, and that something valuable can be done by way of treatment when it is discovered.

We'll look at how these conditions are met by the cervical screening programme and how they relate to the 'big four' cancers – breast, bowel, prostate and lung cancer – and will then touch on the possibility of screening for the types of cancer.

Cervical cancer screening

The cervical screening programme has been running in the UK since the 1980s and is considered a success story. Under the scheme women between the ages of 25 and 64 are asked to go for a test every three years until they are 49 and five-yearly thereafter. In the past this has been the 'smear test', where a wooden spatula is used to scrape a thin layer of cells from the surface of the cervix. The spatula is then slid along a glass slide, leaving a 'smear' of cells which can be stained with special dyes and looked at under the microscope. This is now being replaced by the new technique of liquid-based cytology, where a small brush is used to brush cells from the cervix. The brush is put into a container with special preservative fluid and this then goes to the laboratory for analysis. Liquid-based cytology is slightly more accurate, gives fewer 'uncertain' results (which means fewer repeat tests) and is a bit more comfortable than the older smear test.

If you look at today's figures you may not feel that cervical cancer is that big a problem: each year in the UK there are just under 4,000 new cases diagnosed, and although most of these are cured there are still about 1,400 women who die from the disease ever year. These are relatively small numbers compared to the 'big four'. But the reason the numbers are relatively small is because of the screening programme, which prevents the cancer from developing in the first place. It has been estimated that if it weren't for the screening programme, more than 6,000 women would die annually from cervical cancer in the UK; put another way, cervical screening saves 5,000 lives in the UK every year. So, cervical cancer meets our first condition for successful screening: it is an important health problem.

The second condition is also met: there is a screening test that works, that does what it is supposed to do. For a screening test to be reliable it has to do two things: it has to be sensitive, and it has to be specific. Being sensitive means that it will find a cancer if one is there – it is no good having a test that detects only one in ten of a particular type of cancer and fails to find the other nine. Being specific means that the test is positive for the cancer, but not for other things. To give an example to explain this: some years ago there was great hope that a simple blood test, measuring something called carcino-embryonic antigen, or CEA, could be used to detect bowel cancer. Further research showed that many people with bowel cancer tested positive for CEA, but so did many people with other, non-cancerous, illnesses. A raised CEA level was something that happened in many different diseases – it wasn't specific to bowel cancer. How does the cervical screening test measure up? It does very well: for specificity it scores almost 80 per cent, so it will pick up eight out of ten 'cancers' (I'll explain the inverted commas in a moment). For sensitivity it rates over 90 per cent, so fewer than one in ten tests that appear to be positive will really be due to something other than 'cancer'.

Why the inverted commas in the last paragraph? They were there because although the screening test can pick up cervical cancer, what it most often detects are pre-cancerous changes in the cells on the cervix. These changes are known as either cervical dysplasia or cervical intraepithelial neoplasia (CIN). Over a number of years, if not treated, they will usually progress and turn into cervical cancers. So the screening test usually finds abnormalities in the cells that will lead to cancer some years later, rather than finding established cancers.

Finally, if an abnormality is discovered, can it be treated? The answer is a resounding 'yes'. The changes cervical dysplasia and CIN can be dealt with by minor surgery, which can usually be done as an out-patient or day-patient and will stop a cancer developing. If the screening test has picked up an established cancer, then this will still usually be at a very early stage, where an operation will lead to a cure.

Given all these positives, why do some women still get, and die from, cervical cancer? Well, there is the problem that once every so often the screening test will give a false negative result, that it will say that everything is all clear and miss a cancer. But this is unusual. The bigger problem is that not everybody goes for the screening test. At the present time about 80 per cent or four out every five women who are invited to go for screening actually do so. But this means there are still one in five who don't, and unfortunately the statistics suggest that they are the women who are most likely to be at risk: younger women, in poorer social classes, who are sexually promiscuous. Screening only works if you actually attend for it; it won't protect you if you don't have it.

Breast cancer screening

Breast cancer is a major health problem. About one in nine women will develop the disease at some time during their lives, which means there are more than 40,000 new cases each year in the UK. The good news is that in recent years the cure rate has increased dramatically, so that now more than seven out of ten women who get breast cancer will be cured. But that still means some women won't be so lucky, so screening to detect the disease at its earliest, most curable, stage remains important.

The test used in breast screening is mammography, a breast x-ray. Screening is available for women between the ages of 50 and 70, and is repeated every two years. After 70 you can continue screening if you ask for it, but you won't be sent routine appointments automatically. People often ask why screening isn't offered for younger women. The two main reasons are that breast cancer is much less common in women under 50 – half of all cases occur in women over 65 – and that mammography is much less accurate in younger women, because their breasts are denser and cancers show up less well on the x-rays. However, in the last year or so the NHS has agreed that for young women who are at high risk of developing breast cancer because they have a strong family history of the disease, regular screening can be done using a different test: magnetic resonance imaging, or MRI scanning.

Mammography is a good way of detecting breast cancer in women over 50, but it isn't foolproof. The sensitivity of the test is about 90 per cent and the specificity 95 per cent. That means that it will pick up nine out of ten breast cancers, and that of the tests that are reported positive about one in 20 will turn out to be not a cancer but a benign lesion like scar tissue or a cyst.

As with all medical tests, there will be occasional false negatives and false positives; cancers that are there will be missed, and the test will indicate that something which is harmless is actually a malignant tumour. But as tests go the success rate is pretty good.

The aim of breast screening is to find breast cancers when they are still very small and before they have spread. But the test also often picks up pre-invasive breast cancer, or ductal carcinoma in situ (DCIS). DCIS used to be thought of as a rare condition but it now makes up about a quarter of the cases detected on breast screening. In DCIS, cancer cells are present in the ducts of the breast (the fine tubes that run from the milk glands to the nipple), but have not begun to invade the surrounding breast tissue. Specialists still argue as to whether DCIS is a cancerous or pre-cancerous condition, and there is uncertainty over how often it does turn into an invasive, proper, breast cancer. However, whatever the statistics, with DCIS, as with early breast cancer, simple, relatively minor surgery will get rid of the problem and remove the risk.

Experts estimate that each year in the UK breast screening saves about 1,400 lives. Although most breast cancers can be cured these days, that cure may involve not only surgery but radiotherapy, months of chemotherapy and years of hormone treatment, so picking up the disease before it has really developed, or catching it at its earliest stage when simple surgery will get rid of it, is still very worthwhile. And most women do seem to appreciate this: the take-up rate for breast screening is approaching 80 per cent and increasing every year. So, eight out of ten women who are invited for screening will attend. The main problem here is that many of the 20 per cent of women who don't attend are in ethnic minority populations, and the organizers of the screening programme are making increasing efforts to encourage these ladies to come forward and have their mammograms.

Bowel cancer screening

Bowel cancer, which may be a cancer of either the colon or the rectum, is a major problem. It is the third most common cancer in the UK, with more than 32,000 new cases each year, which means that one in 20 of us will develop the condition at some time during our lives. Treatment usually involves quite major surgery, often followed by chemotherapy and sometimes radiotherapy as well. Despite all this, only about half the people who get bowel cancer are cured. So, trying to prevent the disease, or to catch it at its earliest, most curable stage, is a good idea.

At the present time the Department of Health for England and Wales is rolling out a screening programme for bowel cancer. At the moment this will be limited to people between the ages of 60 and 69 (bowel cancer mainly affects an older age group, although about one in 20 cases, which are caused by inheriting a faulty gene, can occur much earlier in life). The screening test that has been chosen is called the faecal occult blood test (FOB test). This looks for tiny traces of blood in the bowel motions (the stools, or faeces). If traces of blood are found this does not mean that there definitely is a cancer, but it will lead to a further test, called a colonoscopy. The colonoscopy is done at hospital, and involves having a flexible telescope passed up the back passage, so that doctors can look at the bowel and see what caused the bleeding. Sometimes this will be due to non-cancerous causes, like polyps or an inflammation of the bowel, but if a cancer is discovered then it can be treated, and will often be picked up at a very early, curable stage.

With the FOB test people over 60 will automatically be sent a special testing pack in the post. This will tell you how to take samples from three bowel motions and smear these into cards which come with the pack. These can then be hygienically sealed and returned to the laboratory in a Freepost envelope, for testing to see if there is any blood present. It may all sound a bit messy, and a touch embarrassing, but studies have shown that people do actually cope very well with the test, and the kit does come with full instructions. The test is repeated every two years.

The FOB will detect six out of ten bowel cancers. Of those people who have a positive test and go on to have a colonoscopy, about one out of every ten will be found to have a bowel cancer, and about another four out of ten will have a polyp, which could turn into a bowel cancer (this can be removed with a minor operation).

Estimates vary, but figures suggest the introduction of bowel cancer screening could save between 1,200 and 2,000 lives each year in the British Isles.

Prostate cancer

There is no denying that prostate cancer is a major health problem; as we have seen, in the last few years it has become the most common cancer in men in the UK. But there is a difference of opinion between some members of the public and doctors as to the value of screening for the disease. While many people would like to see screening brought in, the medical view is that it would not be very helpful. There are a number of reasons for this.

The screening test for prostate cancer is a simple blood test, called the PSA. This measures an enzyme in the blood called prostate specific antigen, which is raised in many men with prostate cancer. Although it is an easy test the results are not very reliable. It is only about 55 per cent sensitive and 70 per cent specific, so it will fail to detect nearly half of all prostate cancers, and when the test is abnormal this will be due to non-cancerous causes in about one in three cases. So if screening were brought in a lot of men would get false reassurance when a negative test failed to show their cancer, while many others, with a positive test, would go through many unnecessary investigations to show that, in truth, they did not have a cancer.

There is a lot of uncertainty over whether making an early diagnosis is really helpful in prostate cancer. This is because most cases of the disease occur in elderly men, over the age of 75. In this age group prostate cancer usually grows very slowly and often causes few problems, frequently needing little or nothing in the way of treatment. Early diagnosis of a cancer they would otherwise be unaware of, and for which no treatment is needed, could lead to many men having pointless anxiety about having cancer, whereas if they had never had the test they would not have had the worry.

The men who would be most likely to benefit from early discovery of the disease would be those in a younger age group, of

55–65, in whom the cancer can be more aggressive. But prostate cancer at this age is very uncommon, and even with a national screening programme only a handful of cases would be picked up every year. With such a small return the programme would be hopelessly non cost-effective. Although some new cancers would be discovered in younger men, this would be at a cost of hundreds of thousands of pounds every time, and this is something the NHS just can't afford.

Finally, unlike the other cancers we have looked at, there is no very strong evidence that early treatment of prostate cancer actually increases the chance of a cure.

At the present time there are a number of clinical trials underway around the world looking at this question. The early results tend to support the official view that a screening programme would not be worthwhile. Until final, conclusive, evidence is available, the British health authorities have adopted a half-way-house approach to the issue of prostate cancer screening. The current position is that any man over 50 who wants to can ask his GP for a PSA blood test. The GP must then explain the possible benefits and possible disadvantages of the test to him. If, after weighing up the pros and cons, he decides he would like to go ahead, then his GP will arrange the test for him.

Lung cancer

Lung cancer is a major problem, and remains the most common cause of death from cancer in the UK. Smokers, and recent ex-smokers, are an obvious target group for screening because of their increased risk of getting lung cancer. And although ordinary chest x-rays are not very useful as a screening test (they would often only detect the disease when it was quite advanced), a more sophisticated type of imaging, known as a spiral-CT scan, can pick up lung cancers at an early stage. But using these scans as a screening test would be very expensive.

Despite this, there was some encouragement at the end of 2006 when a study in the USA suggested that spiral-CT scans could find very early lung cancers in smokers and ex-smokers, leading to a greatly increased number of operations, which might lead to a cure. But a few months later another study showed that although screening with these scans did find more early cancers, this still did not improve the overall number of cures: just as many people were dying from lung cancer despite the screening.

Further clinical trials are underway, but at the moment the conflicting – and confusing – results from the studies that have been done mean that we are still some way away from having a screening programme for the disease.

Screening in general

There are a few points to remember about screening:

- 'How can I have breast cancer, doctor? My cervical smear test was all clear three months ago.' Over the years, I have regularly heard this in my clinics, and have had to explain that the screening tests we have each look for just one kind of cancer. Cervical screening checks for cervical cancer or pre-cancerous changes in the cervix – it can't check for anything else. So having a negative screening test for one cancer doesn't mean that you can't get another cancer somewhere else in your body.
- Screening tests are regularly repeated, and it is important to have these follow-up tests. Getting the all clear one year doesn't mean that a cancer can't develop a few years later. One negative test is not a lifetime guarantee that you won't get cancer.
- Cancers can appear in between screening tests. But if you do develop one of these 'interval cancers' it will be picked up at an early stage next time and should still be very treatable.

This is another reason for attending regularly when you are offered the chance.

- Cervical screening and bowel screening can both help prevent cancer by detecting conditions which can lead to a cancer developing (CIN in cervical cancer, and polyps in bowel cancer). If a cancer does occur, then breast, cervical and bowel screening will all pick up the great majority of cases in the early stages, when they are still highly treatable and curable.

So the message is, screening is a good thing, and if you are invited to attend for breast or cervical screening, or are sent a bowel cancer screening pack in the post, then do take the opportunity to check that you are all clear – better safe than sorry.

10

It's down to you

This chapter is really a checklist, looking back at the things we have covered in earlier chapters and highlighting the things that each of us can do to reduce our risk of getting cancer.

Lifestyle

Smoking

Smoking, especially cigarette smoking, is a killer. It causes more than nine out of every ten lung cancers and dramatically increases your risk of getting bladder cancer, bowel cancer, cancer of the pancreas and a number of other cancers. None of these is a pleasant disease, and lung and pancreatic cancer in particular have very low cure rates: more than 90 per cent of people who get them will die from them. Prevention definitely is better than cure, especially when there often isn't a cure. If you're a smoker, do try to stop, and chat to your GP or practice nurse about the schemes that are freely available to help you. If you are a non-smoker, then don't even think about starting. And there is the bonus that non-smokers also have a lower risk of serious heart disease and breathing problems.

Watching your weight

Obesity shortens life-expectancy and increases your risk of bowel and kidney cancer; for overweight women, the chances of getting cancer of the womb and breast cancer are increased, and overweight men are more likely to get prostate cancer. And being overweight can lead to potentially fatal heart disease, and to diabetes. So check your height and weight and work out your body mass index (see pp. 51–2). If you find you are in the over-weight or obese range, then seriously think about some dieting to shed the pounds.

Regular exercise

Regular exercise keeps us fit and helps our bodies in many different ways, including keeping our hearts healthy, reducing tiredness and depression, and ensuring our bowels are working well. And active people are less likely to get cancer than people who lead a very sedentary life. You don't have to sign up at the gym and pump iron or do the marathon on the treadmill (though you can if you like). Just a regular brisk half-hour walk five or six times a week is enough to make a difference, and everyday things like using stairs instead of lifts, walking up and down escalators instead of just standing still on them, and walking to the shops or with the kids to school rather than getting the car out.

Eating sensibly

Eating sensibly can also help make a difference. The key things here are plenty of fresh fruit and vegetables: aiming for the government's target of five portions a day is a good starting point. All fruit and vegetables are fine, so there is plenty of choice, but avoid cooking vegetables for too long: the flavour will be better if you don't, and the nutrient content higher. Also, when cooking use olive oil rather than animal fats – many reports have suggested that diets rich in olive oil are healthy, and may even reduce your cancer risk.

Have variety and balance in your diet. If you enjoy red meat, a good steak or roast beef and Yorkshire pudding, then do have them, but no more than once or twice a week, balanced with some white meat, chicken or turkey, and fish. All fresh fish is good, especially oily fish like mackerel and sardines. Be sparing in your intake of processed foods (sausages, pies, pâtés, etc., which often contain a lot of salt, fat and additives) and keep fatty foods and fried foods as occasional treats a few times a week, rather than your routine menu.

Alcohol

If you enjoy a glass of wine, a nip of spirits or a pint of beer, then that's quite OK, but do drink sensibly. Keep within the recommended targets of no more than 14 units a week for a woman and 21 units for a man, remembering that one unit is roughly the same as a small (125 ml) glass of wine, a pint of beer or a single measure of spirits. The argument still goes on, especially in relation to drinking red wine, as to the balance between the risks and benefits to our general health, some studies suggesting that a regular glass of wine actually increases longevity and others being more doubtful. But from a cancer point of view, keeping your drinking within the target levels shouldn't significantly increase your risks, although it could be argued that if you wanted to take every possible precaution against getting the disease then avoiding alcohol completely is the best thing.

Be sun safe

This doesn't mean hiding indoors on beautiful summer days and only going out when it's cloudy or wet. It means being sensible about your exposure to sunlight. The best advice is that of the Sun Smart campaign, which is worth repeating here:

- Avoid going out in the sun between 11 a.m. and 3 p.m., or if you do go out, keep in the shade.
- Make sure you never burn. Sunburn isn't just painful, it doubles your risk of skin cancer.
- If you are going out in strong sunlight cover up with a t-shirt, hat and sunglasses. When the sun is at its peak, sunscreen isn't enough.
- Children should be especially careful; young skin is delicate,

and getting sunburn as a child is even more dangerous than getting it in later life.

- Use a sunscreen with factor 15 or higher, and apply it generously; remember, reapply it often.

Family history: inherited cancers

If one or more close relatives have had cancer, then take a bit of time to make a list of those family members who you know have had the disease, making a note, if you can find this out, of the type of cancer they had and the age at which it was first discovered. If you find you have two or more first-degree relatives with the same type of cancer, or a first-degree relative who had breast or bowel cancer diagnosed at a young age (under 45), or if you are simply worried that there seems to be a lot of cancer in the family, then make your checklist and arrange to see your family doctor and have a chat with him or her, to get advice as to whether or not there might be a problem. The GP will be able to weigh up the risks for you, and either reassure you that the cancers that have occurred in your family are just the result of normal statistical chance, or, if the doctor is suspicious that there could be a genetic cause, a faulty gene running in the family, he or she will be able to make you an appointment with a specialist who can look into things further.

Screening

The earlier a cancer is detected, the more likely it is to be cured. If someone has a bowel cancer that is confined to the inner lining of the bowel then there is a nine out of ten chance that they will be completely cured, but if that cancer is not found until it has spread to the liver the chance of a cure becomes only about one in 20. Similar figures apply for other cancers. In the next year or two, all of us who are over 60 will get invitations to take part in bowel cancer screening, and the screening programmes for breast and cervical cancer are well established. The cervical cancer screening is designed to actually prevent cancer, because it detects changes in the cervix which often predate cancer formation by a number of years, but all three schemes offer a chance of either picking up treatable conditions that might lead to cancer or discover the disease itself at the time when it is most likely to be curable. So if you get invited to have a screening test, do take up the offer – it could be a matter of life or death.

Symptoms

Obsessively checking our bodies three times a day for signs of cancer is not particularly helpful. On the other hand, ignoring symptoms that might be due to cancer, so that a diagnosis and treatment are unnecessarily delayed, can be very harmful. There are a few key symptoms that might mean that you have a cancer, although all of them can be caused by other things as well. The all-important thing is that if you notice one of these problems you don't ignore it or wait for it to get better on its own: you should see your family doctor straight away, to get advice. The key things to look out for are:

- Lumps: if you find a new lump or swelling in any part of your body you should get it checked. Cancerous lumps are often painless in their early stages, so the fact that a lump doesn't hurt doesn't mean it can be ignored.
- Abnormal bleeding: seeing blood in your urine, bleeding from the back passage, coughing up blood or vomiting blood, bleeding from the vagina after the menopause or between periods, can all be signs of underlying cancer. They may be caused by something else, but you should have a check-up to make sure.

- Coughs, breathlessness or hoarseness: all of us get coughs and colds, and these often lead to some shortness of breath, but if you develop these symptoms and they are not getting any better after two weeks you should see your GP. Similarly, if your voice goes hoarse and husky and this hasn't got any better after two weeks, then you should see your family doctor.

- Changes in bowel habit: bleeding from the back passage should always be checked, especially if the blood is dark red rather than bright red – bright red bleeding is most likely to be due to piles (haemorrhoids) but still shouldn't be ignored. If you develop constipation or diarrhoea that goes on for more than a few weeks – say, four to six weeks – without getting better, this also needs attention and advice.

- Moles: all of us have moles, but malignant melanomas are cancerous moles and need urgent attention. The main differences between cancerous and benign moles are: the cancers have irregular edges, whereas benign moles have quite sharply defined margins; cancerous moles are irregular in shape, whereas benign moles tend to be very symmetrical; cancerous moles often have a mix of colours – blue, black, purple, reddish and brown tinges – whereas benign moles are a uniform colour; malignant melanomas tend to be larger than benign moles, so if a mole is more than 7 mm (0.5 in) across then this is suspicious; if an existing mole begins to itch, become crusty or start to bleed, any of these could be a sign that it has become cancerous.

- Unexplained weight loss: if you find you have lost weight over the last couple of months and can't explain this by changes in your diet or taking more exercise, then you should get medical advice, especially if you have feelings of tiredness and are not feeling well.

Get your advice from the right places

Reading the newspapers, browsing the internet, it would be very easy to become extremely confused about what might increase or reduce your chances of getting cancer. Occasionally the information is reliable and helpful, but more often than not it is either reporting early research which needs a lot more work to back it up and prove its worth, or even peddling stories or floating theories that are totally misleading. If there are times when you are puzzled or worried or muddled by things you hear or see in the media or on the web, then the organizations listed in 'Useful addresses' at the end of this book have excellent information services that give very sound advice backed up by leading experts in the field.

The top ten tips

This chapter, and I guess this whole book, can be summarized in the following short checklist of things you can do to help yourself keep your risk of getting cancer to a minimum. The list isn't a guarantee that you won't get the disease – unfortunately, no one can offer that (despite some claims on the internet) – but it offers guidance on how you can tip the odds in your favour:

- Don't smoke; or if you do, stop.
- Watch your weight: if you are overweight, or obese, try to lose weight.
- Exercise regularly.
- Eat sensibly; include plenty of fresh fruit and vegetables in your diet.
- Drink sensibly.
- Be sensible about going out in the sun.
- Be aware of your family medical history, and if you are concerned about the number of cancers see your doctor for further advice.

- Take up invitations for cancer screening programmes.
- Be aware of your body, and if you develop suspicious symptoms see your doctor immediately.
- Get your information about cancer from the right places.

Useful addresses

Cancerbackup
3 Bath Place
Rivington Street
London EC2A 3JR
Tel.: 0808 800 1234 (freephone helpline, UK only)
      020 7739 2280 (standard-rate helpline)
Website: www.cancerbackup.org.uk

Cancerbackup is a comprehensive information service for patients. It offers a telephone helpline to specially trained cancer nurses, who can give advice on all aspects of breast cancer and its treatment. It also produces nearly 70 booklets, and more than 200 factsheets on all aspects of cancer, including breast cancer. There are more than a thousand questions and answers about cancer on its website, and the website also has the texts of all the booklets and factsheets, as well as links to many other useful organizations.

Cancer Research UK
PO Box 123
Lincoln's Inn Fields
London WC2A 3PX
Tel.: 020 7242 0200 (Switchboard)
      020 7121 6699 (Supporter Services)
      0808 800 4040 (Cancer Research UK nurses freephone information
      line)
Website: www.cancerresearchuk.org

As well as funding research on cancer, this organization has an additional website <www.cancerhelp.org.uk>, which gives information about different types of cancer and their treatment, as well as a comprehensive list of clinical trials currently in progress.

DIPEX
Website: www.dipex.org

The initials stand for 'Database of Individual Patient Experiences'. The site covers a number of different illnesses, and has an extensive section on cancer. This not only gives some background information on various types of cancer, but has many stories from people who have had cancer, including breast cancer.

The Health Protection Agency
Central Office
7th Floor, Holborn Gate
330 High Holborn
London WC1V 7PP
Tel.: 020 7759 2700/2701
Website: www.hpa.org.uk

Macmillan Cancer Relief
89 Albert Embankment
London SE1 7UQ
Tel.: 0808 808 2020 (freephone) (CancerLine)
Website: www.macmillan.org.uk

In addition to funding cancer nursing services, this organization provides
a number of publications on breast cancer and a useful booklet on
benefits and financial help for cancer patients. These are all listed on the
website, which also contains useful information on various aspects of
cancer, including a directory of local cancer support groups and patients'
stories about their experiences.

Index